D1545137

Spinal Cord Stimulation

This material is not intended to be, and should not be considered, a substitute for medical or other professional advice. Treatment for the conditions described in this material is highly dependent on the individual circumstances. While this material is designed to offer accurate information with respect to the subject matter covered and to be current as of the time it was written, research and knowledge about medical and health issues is constantly evolving, and dose schedules for medications are being revised continually, with new side effects recognized and accounted for regularly. Readers must therefore always check the product information and clinical procedures with the most up-to-date published product information and data sheets provided by the manufacturers and the most recent codes of conduct and safety regulation. Oxford University Press and the authors make no representations or warranties to readers, express or implied, as to the accuracy or completeness of this material, including without limitation that they make no representations or warranties as to the accuracy or efficacy of the drug dosages mentioned in the material. The authors and the publishers do not accept, and expressly disclaim, any responsibility for any liability, loss, or risk that may be claimed or incurred as a consequence of the use and/or application of any of the contents of this material.

Spinal Cord Stimulation

Percutaneous Implantation Techniques

Paul G. Kreis M.D.
Professor and Medical Director
Division of Pain Medicine
University of California, Davis School of Medicine

Scott M. Fishman M.D.
Professor and Chief
Division of Pain Medicine
University of California, Davis School of Medicine

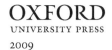

OXFORD
UNIVERSITY PRESS
2009

OXFORD
UNIVERSITY PRESS

Oxford University Press, Inc., publishes works that further
Oxford University's objective of excellence
in research, scholarship, and education.

Oxford   New York
Auckland   Cape Town   Dar es Salaam   Hong Kong   Karachi
Kuala Lumpur   Madrid   Melbourne   Mexico City   Nairobi
New Delhi   Shanghai   Taipei   Toronto

With offices in
Argentina   Austria   Brazil   Chile   Czech   Republic France   Greece
Guatemala   Hungary   Italy   Japan   Poland   Portugal   Singapore
South Korea   Switzerland   Thailand   Turkey   Ukraine   Vietnam

Copyright © 2009 by the authors.

Published by Oxford University Press, Inc.
198 Madison Avenue, New York, New York 10016
www.oup.com

Oxford is a registered trademark of Oxford University Press

All rights reserved. No part of this publication may be reproduced,
stored in a retrieval system, or transmitted, in any form or by any means,
electronic, mechanical, photocopying, recording, or otherwise,
without the prior permission of the authors.

Library of Congress Cataloging-in-Publication Data

Kreis, Paul.
  Spinal cord stimulation : percutaneous implantation techniques / Paul Kreis, Scott Fishman.
    p. ; cm.
  Includes bibliographical references and index.
  ISBN 978-0-19-539365-1
1. Transcutaneous electrical nerve stimulation. 2. Spinal cord. 3. Implants, Artificial. I. Fishman, Scott, 1959- II. Title.
  [DNLM: 1. Electric Stimulation Therapy—methods. 2. Neuralgia—surgery. 3. Electrodes, Implanted.
4. Spinal Cord—physiology. 5. Spinal Cord—radiation effects. WL 544 K92s 2009]
  RM880.K74 2009
  617.4'82—dc22   2008055855

Manuscript development was supported by an unrestricted educational grant from Boston Scientific Neuromodulation.

Paul G. Kreis has served as a consultant to Boston Scientific Neuromodulation.
Scott M. Fishman has nothing to disclose.

Preface

Spinal cord stimulation (SCS) was introduced in 1967 as a neurosurgical treatment for otherwise intractable pain.[1] Compared with alternative surgical procedures for pain, SCS is less invasive and less disruptive because it does not ablate pain pathways or result in anatomic change. As an augmentative procedure, SCS is reversible and offers patients the opportunity of undergoing a screening trial with a temporary SCS system before proceeding (or not) to implantation. This screening trial emulates the results of the implantation exactly and, thus, provides an advantage not shared by anatomic (e.g., bracing to predict response to spinal fusion) or ablative prognostic procedures (e.g., reversible local anesthetic blockade to predict response to nerve section).

In the 1970s, clinicians developed a minimally invasive percutaneous method of inserting temporary catheter electrodes for use in the SCS screening trial, with the expectation that permanent plate/paddle electrode implantation would occur via laminectomy.[2,3] Soon thereafter, adoption of these percutaneous techniques for permanent implantation yielded results approaching those achieved with surgical techniques.[4] Indeed, the majority of SCS procedures are performed by physicians who are not surgeons and must rely on use of percutaneous electrodes. These clinicians will find this book especially pertinent and helpful, as its contents range from a presentation of the fundamentals of SCS to an overview of basic surgical principles. Of course no book, no matter how thoughtful, is a substitute for clinical training and hands-on experience, but this volume meets an important need and will be a valuable resource for practitioners of SCS.

When SCS is delivered to the right (properly selected) patient by the right (experienced) clinician in the right setting using the right equipment and technique, results are optimized, and relief of otherwise intractable pain can be sustained for decades. Therefore, it is not surprising that ongoing improvement in these variables has led to an increasing body of high-quality medical evidence indicating that in selected patients the result of SCS treatment for neuropathic pain is superior to that achieved with surgical[5] or medical[6] treatment. Resources such as this book will help enhance the quality of SCS treatment and improve patient outcomes as SCS becomes more widely available.

Richard B. North, MD
LifeBridge Brain & Spine Institute, Baltimore, MD
Professor of Neurosurgery, Anesthesiology and
Critical Care Medicine (retired)
Johns Hopkins University School of Medicine

REFERENCES

1. Shealy CN, Mortimer JT, Reswick JB. Electrical inhibition of pain by stimulation of the dorsal columns: preliminary clinical report. *Anesth Analg* 1967;46(4):489–91.
2. Erickson DL. Percutaneous trial of stimulation for patient selection for implantable stimulating devices. *J Neurosurg* 1975;34:440–4.
3. Hosobuchi Y, Adams JE, Weinstein PR. Preliminary percutaneous dorsal column stimulation prior to permanent implantation. *J Neurosurg* 1972;17:242–5.
4. North RB, Fischell TA, Long DM. Chronic stimulation via percutaneously inserted epidural electrodes. *Neurosurgery* 1977;1(2):215–8.
5. North RB, Kidd DH, Farrokhi F, et al. Spinal cord stimulation versus repeated lumbosacral spine surgery for chronic pain: a randomized, controlled trial. *Neurosurgery* 2005;56(1):98–106.
6. Kumar K, Taylor RS, Jacques L, et al. Spinal cord stimulation versus conventional medical management for neuropathic pain: a multicentre randomised controlled trial in patients with failed back surgery syndrome. *Pain* 2007;132(1–2):179–88.

Acknowledgments

This book is a synthesis of decades of experience, research, and wisdom based on the work of countless individuals to whom we are truly grateful. I am particularly indebted to several gifted friends and mentors who have inspired me, guided me, and believed in me.

First, I would like to sincerely thank my wife Terrie and my daughters Lauren, and Rachel for being so understanding and patient during the summer of 2007 when I was largely unavailable. Your love and support continue to inspire me.

Next, I would like to thank my dear friend, mentor, role model, and partner, Scott Fishman, without whom, this book would never have come to print. Not only did Scott contribute as a co-author, but he anticipated in advance every possible contingency and skillfully helped guide me through each challenge that arose. His unwavering energy, enthusiastic encouragement and advice from beginning to end were instrumental in taking this project to completion.

I would also like to thank Dr. Kenneth M. Alo, MD for his thoughtful and thorough review of the entire text. I can't say enough about Dr. Alo's vast experience, contribution to the literature, and commitment to the field of neuromodulation. He has been and continues to be an inspiration to me.

I would like to sincerely thank Dr. James J. Chao, MD who critically and meticulously reviewed the surgical chapters. His expertise as a plastic surgeon and his constructive teaching style have made this a much better book and me a much better implanter.

I would like to personally thank Peter Moore, MD, chair of the anesthesiology department at the University of California, Davis. His unwavering support for the mission of the division of pain medicine has created the foundation for projects like this as well as many others.

I would like to recognize the contribution of my father, Van Allen Kreis, MD who read and edited each chapter of this text with remarkable skill, insight, and thoughtfulness. Thanks so much for a lifetime of support and encouragement.

I was privileged to have Kerry Bradley, a brilliant and widely published expert on the technology of neuromodulation, review and edit the chapter on electricity and spinal cord stimulation. This was undoubtedly one of the more complex chapters, and I am very grateful to Kerry for his in-depth review.

A special thanks to my long-time friend and colleague, Brian Moffit, MD for his review of the chapter on Radiation Safety.

Many thanks to Katherine Chau for taking on and completing the daunting task of organizing the references.

I would like to thank Ethan Covey, Peter Hurwitz, John Lappola and Wendy Kopf for their expertise, professionalism, and commitment to the development of the manuscript. What a great team.

Last I would like to thank Tim Adams, Allen Meacham, and Mike Onuscheck who, more than two years ago said, "You know, you really should write a book." Well, here it is.

—Paul G. Kreis M.D.

It was a pleasure and honor to help Paul Kreis produce this book. He is a pillar of our pain program at UC Davis, a remarkably talented physician, my professional partner and dear friend. This book is his creation and reflects his deep understanding and passion for spinal cord stimulators. He has helped me advance my career and graciously allowed me to help with this project.

I am blessed with a wonderful family who allow me to focus on my work and support me in all ways. I must thank my wonderful wife Blanca and my children Lucas and Elsa who sacrifice for my work and give me great joy. I also must thank my professional family at the UC Davis Division of Pain Medicine. They support my work and provide a professional community that is rare and much appreciated. In particular, I must thank Drs. Gagan Mahajan, Ken Furukawa, Lana Wania Galicia, Aida Phelan, Ingela Symreng, Barth Wilsey, Jack MacMillan, and Mark Holtsman. I also thank Dr. Peter Moore who leads our department of anesthesiology. He has supported Paul Kreis and me personally and has been the guiding force behind pain medicine at UC Davis.

There are many individuals who helped produce this book to whom we are most grateful – Paul Kreis has mentioned most of them in his note. Last but not least, I'd like to thank Yvonne Honigsberg at Oxford University Press who took care of all the details of bringing this book to press, and pushed it on to publication.

The sections entitled "Further Reading" at the end of Chapter 1 (pgs 8–9), Chapter 2 (pgs 20–27, with the exception of the first 5 citations under "Pain Map"), Chapter 5 (pgs 61–62), Chapter 6 (pg 68, with the exception of the first 3 citations), Chapter 8 (pgs 92–93), and Chapter 12 (pgs 141–145) are reproduced from North R and Shipley J: Practice parameters for the use of spinal cord stimulation in the treatment of chronic neuropathic pain. *Pain Med* 2007:8(4):S200–275. We are grateful to these authors. For additional information, please visit the website for the Neuromodulation Foundation at http://www.neuromodfound.org.

—Scott M. Fishman M.D.

Contents

1

The Development of Spinal Cord Stimulation

Introduction

Chronic pain is a substantial medical problem in the United States. At any given time, approximately 9% of U.S. adults experience moderate to severe non–cancer-related pain, which results in some 515 million lost days of work and 40 million physician visits each year. The estimated annual economic losses attributed to chronic pain exceed $100 billion.[1]

Spinal cord stimulation (SCS) is a well-established, reversible therapy for certain types of chronic, neuropathic pain. Successful implantation of an SCS system can result in pain relief, reduced utilization of health care resources, increased activities of daily living, and reduced medication requirement, potentially leading to improved neurologic and cognitive functioning. SCS involves placing stimulator leads into the epidural space and surgically implanting a programmable pulse generator subcutaneously. Although the surgery is relatively minor, it requires specialized training and experience to perform safely and effectively. Part of such training is gaining an understanding of the technology, its appropriate applications, and its limitations. Additionally, the surgical techniques involved in implantation must be understood and mastered before the procedure is performed.

To date, there has been no single source of information detailing the skills and techniques necessary to perform SCS. Although the information is available, it is dispersed throughout the literature of several disciplines, including pain medicine, anesthesiology, neurosurgery, radiology, as well as psychology, and includes disparate techniques and management strategies that are found in divergent fields such as surgery or infection control. Thus, this volume offers an introduction to percutaneous SCS and brings together current information from these various sources. It should not be considered an exhaustive text. The focus is primarily on techniques of implanting the stimulator leads and pulse generator, but we do not address surgical paddle lead implantation. Some relevant background information has been provided to put the rest of the volume in context,

and the references provide more definitive sources of information and technique. A thorough understanding of the information presented here should prepare readers for more formal hands-on training.

This book is not intended to take the place of formal training and mentoring. Every prospective implanter should participate in thorough formal training with a respected and experienced surgeon before placing an SCS in a live patient. We believe that having several mentors is probably best so that novice implanters can arrive at a technique that works best for them.

History

Sensory stimulation has been used to treat pain since antiquity.[2] It is believed that ancient Egyptians may have used electrogenic fish to treat ailments 4,500 years ago.[3] One such fish, the black torpedo fish, was used for centuries by the ancient Greeks and Romans (Fig. 1.1).

The live fish was placed over the painful site, and the patient endured the electrical discharge from the fish until the pain was relieved. The Roman physician Scribonius Largus[4] recorded the medical use of the torpedo fish in 46 CE,[3] and Claudius Galen (131–201 CE) also described shocks from the torpedo fish to treat gout and headache.[5]

An 1871 publication by Beard and Rockwell[6] presented a case of "Faradization" and described the application of faradic current (i.e., discontinuous, asymmetric, alternating current) to stimulate muscles and nerves in a subject using a direct current inductorium device (Figs. 1.2a & b). Units such as that shown in Figure 1.3 were also used by early researchers, including Benjamin Franklin, for pain relief, as well as for treatment of other ailments.

The first modern attempt at electrical stimulation of the brain took place in a conscious patient in 1874. The patient had osteomyelitis of the scalp, and the brain was exposed during débridement. Muscle contractions were apparent when

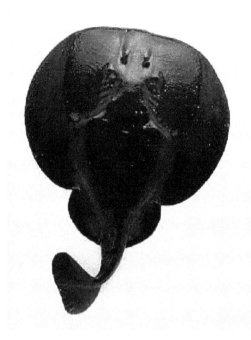

Figure 1.1 The black torpedo fish. Reprinted with permission from www.dkimages.com and Pearson Photography Agency.

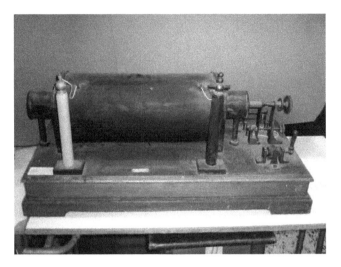

Figure 1.3 Inductorium device. Reprinted with permission from the Science and Technology Museum, University Junior College, Physics Department, Malta.

the exposed motor cortex was subjected to electrical stimulation but not when it was mechanically stimulated.[7] Not until 1948, however, were electrodes successfully implanted in the brain, to treat a patient with a psychiatric disorder.

The Electreat, the first electrical stimulator designed specifically for therapeutic use, was patented by Charles Willie Kent in 1919. It appears to have been remarkably similar to transcutaneous electrical nerve stimulation units that would appear later in the century (Fig. 1.4).

Advertised to the public as a cure-all therapy, an estimated 250,000 Electreat stimulators were sold over the next 25 years. Eventually, Kent would be the first individual prosecuted under the new 1938 Food, Drug, and Cosmetic Act for making unsubstantiated medical claims for the device. The Electreat Company was subsequently forced to limit its claims to pain relief alone.

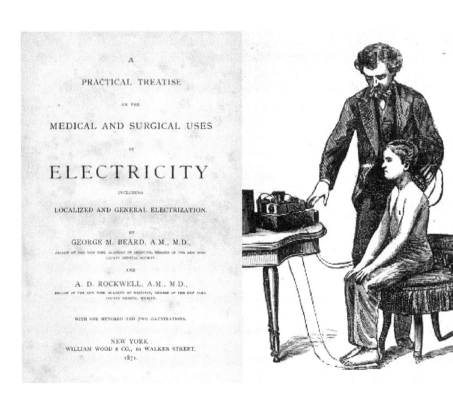

Figure 1.2 *A Practical Treatise on Medical Electricity.* Beard, an early American neurologist, was the first to publish in the field of the medical use of electricity. Rockwell is probably best known for designing the electric chair. Beard GM, Rockwell AD. *A practical treatise on the medical and surgical uses of electricity.* New York:1871. Copyright 2000–2008, The Burton Report®, All rights reserved. www.burtonreport.com.

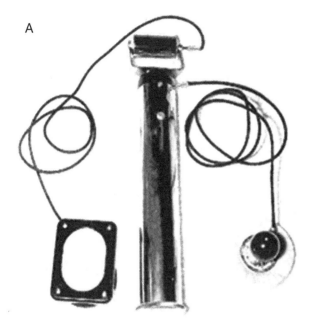

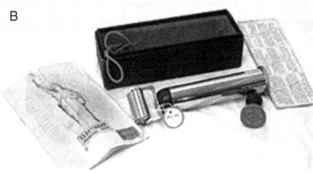

Figure 1.4 (A) The Electreat. The Electreat patented by Charles Willie Kent in 1919. Copyright 2000-2008, The Burton Report®, All rights reserved. www.burtonreport.com. (B) The Electreat Faradaic coil with books. http://www.thebakken. org/artifacts/database/artifact.asp?type=category&category=C2.2&id =1385 Reprinted with permission from The Bakken Library and Museum.

The Gate Theory of Pain Reduction

It has been recognized for years that the perception of pain is not simply proportional to the intensity of the stimulus, but is somehow modulated by higher neuronal centers. This has repeatedly been seen in combat situations where soldiers, following acute injury, initially exhibit no signs of pain and in many cases do not realize that they have been seriously injured until much later.

In 1965, Ron Melzack and Patrick Wall published their gate control theory of pain reduction, which ultimately led to the development of SCS.[8] Gate theory suggests that pain is a complex neurologic and perceptual phenomenon. It postulates that pain perception is a function of the balance between the impulses transmitted to the spinal cord through both the

larger myelinated nerve fibers and the smaller pain fibers, both of which synapse at the dorsal horn. Although still providing a partial explanation after more than 40 years, the exact details of gate theory have been challenged for their accuracy. Neuromodulation of pain is more complex than originally believed, and other mechanisms not explained by gate theory are most certainly involved. For instance, direct inhibition of pain transmission in the dorsal horn of the spinal cord cannot fully explain the mechanism of action of SCS. If direct inhibition were the principal mechanism of action, SCS would also control nociceptive pain, and this is not supported by clinical experience.[2] Additionally, we observe that many patients continue to experience pain relief for many hours after the SCS pulse generator is turned off. Despite its oversimplification, gate theory continues to provide a useful operational framework for the way in which SCS exerts its effect on pain.

Three types of pain are generally recognized today: nociceptive, neuropathic, and idiopathic. *Nociceptive pain* is produced when specialized sensory receptors, called nociceptors, are activated by noxious stimuli. In contrast, *neuropathic pain* is produced only when the nerve cells in either the central or peripheral nervous systems are themselves damaged or dysfunctional. *Idiopathic pain* is simply pain that cannot be explained by either of the other two mechanisms.

Several types of nociceptors have been identified: thermal, mechanical, and chemical. Some nociceptors respond to more than one of these stimuli and are consequently designated *polymodal* nociceptors. Pain signals received from nociceptors are transmitted via afferent *A-delta* and *C-fibers* to the dorsal horn. A-delta fibers are composed of medium-diameter, lightly myelinated axons, and C-fibers are composed of small-diameter, nonmyelinated axons. A-delta nerve fibers transmit pain signals to the spinal cord at approximately 40 mph, whereas C-fibers transmit pain signals at approximately 3 mph. Thus, the sensation of acute, nociceptive pain that is felt immediately after injury is transmitted by A-delta fibers, and the delayed, noxious, deep aching sensation occurring a few seconds later is thought to be transmitted by C-fibers.

Gate theory postulates that signals from the large A-beta sensory and smaller A-delta and C-fibers compete for passage through a physiologic "gate." Only one type of signal can pass through the gate at a time. An increase in large nerve-fiber activity could, through interneurons (nerve cells found within the dorsal horn of the spinal cord that act as links between peripheral neurons and central neurons) potentially "close the gate" to signals from small pain fibers entering the dorsal horn. Closing the gate halts the transmission of pain signals to the brain from these small-diameter fibers. Theoretically, that is why rubbing the skin over an acute blunt injury seems to mitigate pain. Melzack and Wall believed that preferential electrical stimulation of A-beta fibers would "close the gate" to pain transmission and reduce the number of pain signals transmitted to the brain (Fig. 1.5).[8]

Clinical support for gate theory came in 1967, when C. Norman Shealy, a Harvard-trained neurosurgeon at Case Western Reserve University, implanted the first unipolar SCS.[4]

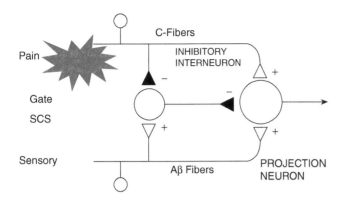

Figure 1.5 Diagram of the gate theory as postulated by Melzack and Wall. Reprinted with permission from Melzack R, Wall PD. Pain mechanisms: a new theory. *Science* 1965;150:171–9.

The stimulator was placed in the intrathecal space adjacent to the dorsal column of the spinal cord in a patient with terminal cancer and neuropathic pain. Considering the potential for mishap, it is remarkable that not only was the surgery technically successful but the patient also experienced marked pain reduction.

In 1973, Hosobuchi reported the first application of deep brain stimulation for treating neuropathic facial pain. Over the next several years, neuromodulation of the central nervous system (CNS) was used only sporadically because of frequent complications. Nonetheless, publications documenting the use of SCS for treating seizure disorders, movement disorders, and spasticity began to appear in the medical literature. In 1984, the effect of SCS on angina was reported as a chance finding in a patient who had a stimulator implanted for another reason.[7] SCS systems were first implanted specifically for intractable angina in Australia in 1987.

Advances in cardiac pacemaker technology led to the development of implantable pulse generators in the mid-1980s, followed by dual multipolar leads and resulting in more effective and reliable systems. Since that time, SCS systems have become much more refined and technologically advanced.

Mechanism of Action

Our understanding of the mechanisms underlying SCS is still in its early stages and is far from being fully elucidated. A better understanding of how SCS modulates the nervous system is needed to perfect and expand current applications. The mechanisms of SCS probably differ depending on the type of pain that is being treated. For example, its effect on neuropathic pain may be secondary to stimulation-induced suppression of central excitability, whereas its effect on ischemic pain may be due to stimulation-induced inhibition of sympathetic outflow and antidromic vasodilation, which increases blood flow to the ischemic area and decreases oxygen demand (Fig. 1.6).[9]

Figure 1.6 Spinal cord stimulation. Spinal cord stimulation (SCS) activates the dorsal columns (DC) orthodromically and antidromically (green lightning bolt). The antidromic activity is transmitted into the dorsal horns (DHs) via DC collaterals. In the DHs, it activates inhibitory circuits (GABAergic, etc.); this acts on the hyperexcitable DH neurons to decrease the high level of the excitatory amino acids (e.g., glutamate. Furthermore, activity ascending from the SCS may activate a supraspinal neuronal loop that induces inhibition from descending pathways, possibly utilizing 5-HT and norepinephrine as transmitters. *WDR, wide-dynamic range; GABA, gamma-aminobutyric acid.* Reprinted from Linderoth B, Foreman RD. Mechanisms of spinal cord stimulation in painful syndromes: role of animal models. *Pain Med* 2006;7(suppl 1): S14–26. With permission from Blackwell Publishing.

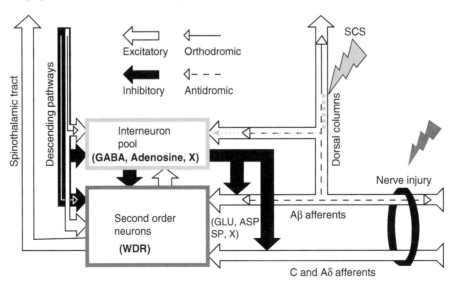

Unfortunately, because the precise neurophysiology of neuropathic pain is not completely understood, the mechanisms underlying the actions of SCS are likewise not known with certainty (Fig. 1.7). Observation of SCS in animal models of neuropathic pain has led to the following possible mechanisms:

- SCS (in animals) attenuates the response to nerve injury in which wide-dynamic-range neurons in the dorsal horn become hyperexcitable and glutamate and gamma-aminobutyric acid (GABA) levels increase and decrease respectively.
- SCS effects appear to be segmental, although supraspinal descending inhibition may be involved through release of serotonin and norepinephrine.
- GABA-B activation by SCS leads to a decrease in glutamate release in the dorsal horn of rats.
- SCS-induced analgesia appears to be resistant to naloxone reversal, suggesting minimal if any involvement of the opioid system.

In most neuropathic pain states, a paresthesia or tingling sensation must be felt in the affected area for SCS to be effective. In patients with deafferentation or CNS damage, such as brachial plexus avulsion or complete spinal cord injury, it is impossible to produce a paresthesia because the necessary neuronal structures have been damaged. SCS will therefore be ineffective in these situations.

The mechanism of action for SCS in ischemic pain is believed to be somewhat different from that of neuropathic pain. In ischemia, SCS appears to increase and redistribute blood flow to the ischemic area as well as decrease tissue oxygen demand. The mechanism by which SCS relieves ischemic pain is thought to involve suppression of the efferent sympathetic activity, resulting in a decrease in peripheral vasoconstriction and relief of pain; and activation of the antidromic mechanisms below the motor threshold, which may result in the release of peripheral calcitonin gene-related peptide with subsequent peripheral vasodilatation.[10]

Equipment Overview

Today, an SCS system consists of an *epidural lead* or *leads,* each containing multiple stimulating *electrodes.* The leads can be one of two types: percutaneous or surgical paddle leads. Percutaneous leads, introduced in the 1970s, are cylindrical insulated catheters with multiple stimulating electrodes spaced sequentially near the distal end. Surgical paddle leads are flat, with an insulated backing that forces current to flow anteriorly toward the dorsal columns; a laminotomy is required for placement. The leads are connected to a *pulse generator* either directly or via an extension. The pulse generator contains the battery and programmable elements of the system. Implantation is a surgical procedure requiring an operating room, surgical and aseptic technique, and prophylactic antibiotics. In addition to the stimulator leads, a standard lead kit also contains a Tuohy needle, lead stylets, guidewire, tunneling tools, lead anchors, and a screening cable (Figs. 1.8a & b).

One of the major advantages to SCS is that a trial of stimulation can be conducted that replicates the permanent implantation. During the trial, leads are placed percutaneously and connected to an external pulse generator. The electrodes used in a percutaneous trial will be removed after the trial, and new electrodes will be implanted with the pulse generator in the permanent implantation. Alternatively, the leads used in a successful tunneled trial will be left in place and connected to a pulse generator for permanent implantation.

During an SCS trial, with the patient under local anesthesia and prone in a fluoroscopy procedure suite, a Tuohy needle (Fig. 1.9) is placed epidurally using a paramedian oblique approach (Figs. 1.10a & b).

An electrode is then threaded through the needle and positioned at the appropriate level under fluoroscopic guidance. The electrode is then attached to the external pulse generator, which produces paresthesia sensations. The correct position of the electrode is determined when the area of paresthesia matches the distribution of pain. If pain is markedly reduced during the trial period, which usually ranges from 3 to 8 days, permanent implantation is subsequently scheduled.

In a permanent trial (see Chapter 8) or a permanent implantation procedure (see Chapter 10), the procedure is performed in the operating room under local anesthesia and conscious sedation. The pulse generator is placed subcutaneously in a comfortable location that is determined before the procedure. Leads placed in the epidural space are then tunneled under the skin either to the pulse generator directly or via an extension lead.

Figure 1.7 Effects of spinal cord stimulation (SCS) on the L1–L2 dorsal columns. SCS activates interneurons that may 1) reduce the activity of spinothalamic tract (STT) cells; 2) decrease the activity of sympathetic preganglionic neurons; 3) reduce the release of norepinephrine from sympathetic postganglionic neurons; 4) activate antidromically the dorsal root afferent fibers; and 5) release calcitonin gene-related peptide (CGRP) and nitric oxide (NO). Reprinted from Linderoth B, Foreman RD. Mechanisms of spinal cord stimulation in painful syndromes: role of animal models. *Pain Med* 2006;7(suppl 1):S14–26. With permission from Blackwell Publishing.

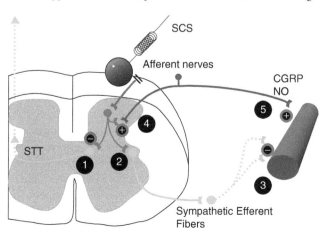

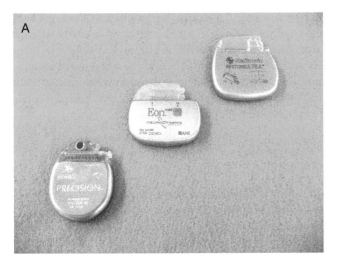

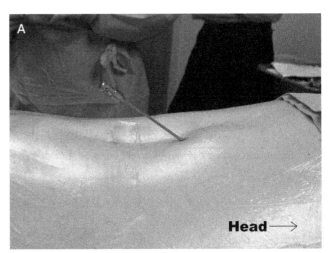

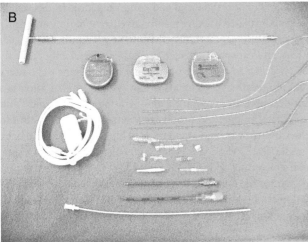

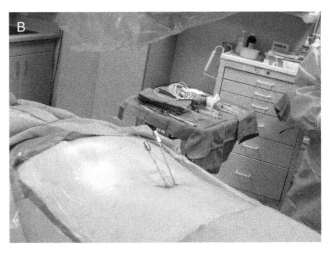

Figure 1.10 Tuohy needle at correct angle of entry.

Figure 1.8 Batteries and equipment. Reprinted with permission from ©2009 Boston Scientific, Inc., St. Jude Medical, Inc., and Medtronic., Inc.

Current Status

SCS technology has evolved impressively over the past 20 years. Stimulator leads have become smaller and more maneuverable, which makes them easier to steer within the epidural space. The leads now contain more electrodes for greater programming options, including reprogramming in the event of minor lead migration. Pulse generator technology has advanced as well.

Figure 1.9 Tuohy needle and stylet.

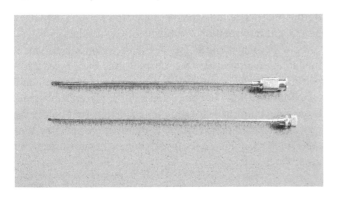

Implanted pulse generators have become smaller, with much greater programming capabilities. The U.S. Food and Drug Administration (FDA) has recently approved rechargeable batteries that last many years.

As the technology has advanced, novel applications for SCS are being explored, such as stimulation to treat ischemic pain (including angina), stimulation of the spinal nerve roots, and peripheral nerve stimulation (see Chapter 2).

Today, SCS is a long-term treatment for a chronic pain condition and thus requires an appropriate infrastructure for surveillance and support.[2] Although SCS is minimally invasive and reversible and does not change a patient's anatomy—in contrast to spine surgery or nerve ablation—it should still be offered only by facilities that can perform comprehensive pain assessments and a wide range of additional interventional, pharmacologic, and psychological therapy.[2] Additionally, permanent SCS systems must be implanted in an appropriately equipped operating room, with anesthesia and postanesthesia care readily available.[2] A multidisciplinary pain management team is also desirable.[2] SCS may be used with other therapies and should be part of an overall rehabilitation strategy.[2]

Favorable Patient Characteristics

Chapter 2 details criteria for patient selection. Current data suggest that, when SCS is indicated, it is more likely to be successful in patients who have:

- Neuropathic pain, not nociceptive pain[11]
- Anatomically limited pain, rather than diffuse pain syndromes[11]
- Unilateral, not bilateral, pain[11]
- Radicular, not central, pain[11]
- Nonmalignant pain[12]
- Poor response to conservative treatment for at least 6 months[12]
- Contraindications for remedial surgery[12]
- No major psychiatric disorders, including somatization disorder[12]
- No history of illicit drug use[12]
- No secondary gain or pending litigation for their condition[12]
- A successful 3- to 8-day screening trial of SCS. (Historically, it has been recommended that patients reporting at least a 50% reduction in pain scores during the trial be considered for permanent SCS.)

Chapter 2 also details cautions, indications, and contraindications for SCS.

Efficacy

The efficacy of SCS has been well documented in the literature over the past 40 years, especially for neuropathic low back and leg pain. More than 500 clinical trials, 38 of them randomized controlled trials, have been conducted on SCS since 1973. The most common end points used in efficacy studies are:

- Reduction in pain intensity, as measured on a 10-cm visual analog scale (VAS); typically, a 50% reduction from pretreatment VAS scores is required to establish efficacy.
- Decreased use of pain medications
- Improved function scores
- Improved activities of daily living (ADL) scores
- Improved quality-of-life scores
- Return to work
- Confirmation that the patient would again choose SCS

By these criteria, success rates of 50% to 70% are common. A systematic review of SCS used to treat failed back surgery syndrome (FBSS) found that on average, almost 60% of patients reported at least a 50% reduction in pain.[13] Other studies have reported 40% to 80% reductions in the use of pain medicines, 61% improvements in ADLs, and 25% return-to-work rates.[7]

In general, SCS appears to be effective primarily in treating neuropathic pain syndromes. In particular, neuropathic leg pain and complex regional pain syndrome (CRPS) respond well to SCS. Cameron, in a systematic review of studies published between 1981 and 2001, grouped success rates by diagnosis. Among the 49 studies reporting long-term results (more

than 6 months of follow-up), success rates ranged from 57% for patients with back and leg pain (the most common indication) to 83% for patients with CRPS (the next most common indication).[14] Additionally, the success rate was 67% in patients with FBSS, stump pain, or peripheral neuropathy, 77% in patients with ischemic limb pain, and 82% in patients with postherpetic neuralgia.[14]

There is no conclusive evidence that SCS is effective in treating nociceptive pain unless it is secondary to ischemia. SCS also appears to be more effective in treating extremity or radicular pain than axial, midline pain even when the axial pain is neuropathic, which is common after back surgery.

As promising as SCS has become, 20% to 40% of patients report loss of analgesia within 24 months of implantation.[15] Growing anecdotal evidence suggests that when this loss of analgesia occurs, it can often be remedied by reimplantation of a new pulse generator with more robust programming capabilities. Further study is necessary to confirm these observations.

Cost-Effectiveness

SCS is a cost-effective treatment for neuropathic pain.[1,2,16] In a meta-analysis of 14 studies across a range of indications, the treatment costs of SCS were consistently offset by reductions in post-implant healthcare costs.[16]

Costs associated with SCS can be divided into initial implantation costs, which include the cost of the SCS implant and hospital stay, and maintenance costs, which include any revisions, physician visits, and electrode and battery replacements. The variation in these costs among the 14 studies was considerable but was offset by savings in all studies after a period ranging from 15 months to 5 years. The critical factors in determining the length of implant time required for the cost of SCS to be offset by savings were the degree of efficacy, duration of battery and electrode life, and level of use by the patient.[16] In a retrospective study of 222 consecutive patients treated with either SCS or peripheral nerve stimulation at the Cleveland Clinic in Ohio, Mekhail et al. reported similar findings. Although the initial implantation costs were high, they were offset by reductions in the number of office visits, nerve blocks, imaging studies, emergency room visits, hospitalizations, and surgical procedures. Costs for the initial two-stage SCS implantation procedure averaged $24,130 over 50 patients in the Cleveland Clinic study and ranged from $14,296 to $34,000 in the studies included in the meta-analysis, some of which were conducted in countries other than the United States. The mean savings per patient was approximately $30,000 per year and more than $90,000 per patient over the 3-year average follow-up period.[1]

Warnings

Physicians and patients engaging in SCS implantation must be aware of the following limitations and features of SCS technology:

- Safety has not been established for pregnant women or for children.

- Patients should not drive or operate dangerous or heavy equipment during stimulation.
- Patients should avoid exposure to magnetic resonance imaging, diathermy, and electrocautery, as electrical energy can be induced through the implant, causing damage to the device, electrodes, and surrounding tissue, resulting in severe injury or even death. Patients should use caution when exposed to ultrasonic equipment, radiation therapy, aircraft communication systems, and other sources of strong electromagnetic interference, as there is a potential for interaction. The device manufacturer can provide additional details on the risks and recommendations if exposure to these devices is necessary.
- Patients should not scuba dive deeper than 10 meters or sustain pressures in a hyperbaric chamber above 2 atmosphere absolute (ATA).

REFERENCES

1. Mekhail NA, Aeschbach A, Stanton-Hicks M. Cost benefit analysis of neurostimulation for chronic pain. *Clin J Pain* 2004;20: 462–8.
2. British Pain Society. *Spinal cord stimulation for the management of pain: recommendations for best clinical practice.* London: British Pain Society, 2005.
3. Kane K, Taub A. A history of local electrical analgesia. *Pain* 1975; 1:25–138.
4. Rossi U. The history of electrical stimulation of the nervous system for the control of pain. In: Simpson BA, ed. *Electrical stimulation and the relief of pain: pain research and clinical management,* Vol. 15. New York: Elsevier Science; 2003:5–16.
5. Stillings D. A survey of the history of electrical stimulation for pain to 1900. *Medical Instrum* 1975;9:255–9.
6. Beard GM, Rockwell AD. *A practical treatise on the medical and surgical uses of electricity.* New York: 1871.
7. Gildenberg PL. History of electrical neuromodulation for chronic pain. *Pain Med* 2006;7(suppl 1):S7–13.
8. Melzack R, Wall PD. Pain mechanisms: a new theory. *Science* 1965;150:171–9.
9. Linderoth B, Foreman RD. Mechanisms of spinal cord stimulation in painful syndromes: role of animal models. *Pain Med* 2006; 7(suppl 1):S14–26.
10. Stojanovic MP, Abdi S. Spinal cord stimulation. *Pain Physician* 2002;5:156–66.
11. North RB, Wetzel FT. Spinal cord stimulation for chronic pain of spinal origin: a valuable long-term solution. *Spine* 2002;27: 2584–92.
12. Lee AW, Pilitsis JG. Spinal cord stimulation: indications and outcomes. *Neurosurg Focus* 2006;21:E3.
13. Turner JA, Loeser JD, Bell KG. Spinal cord stimulation for chronic low back pain: a systematic literature synthesis. *Neurosurgery* 1995; 37:1088–96.
14. Cameron T. Safety and efficacy of spinal cord stimulation for the treatment of chronic pain: a 20-year literature review. *J Neurosurg* 2004;100(suppl):254–67.
15. Doleys D. Psychological factors in spinal cord stimulation therapy: brief review and discussion. *Neurosurg Focus* 2006; 21:1–6.
16. Taylor RS, Taylor RJ, Van Buyten JP, et al. The cost effectiveness of spinal cord stimulation in the treatment of pain: a systematic review of the literature. *J Pain Symptom Manage* 2004;27:370–8.

Further Reading

Cost-Effectiveness of SCS for FBSS

Estimates of Annual Costs of Nonsurgical Treatment

Bell GK, Kidd D, North RB. Cost-effectiveness analysis of spinal cord stimulation in treatment of failed back surgery syndrome. *J Pain Symptom Manage* 1997;13:286–95.
de Lissovoy G, Brown RE, Halpern M, et al. Cost effectiveness of long-term intrathecal morphine for pain associated with failed back syndrome. *Clin Ther* 1997;19:96–112.
Luo X, Pietrobon R, Sun SX, et al. Estimates and patterns of direct health care expenditures among individuals with back pain in the United States. *Spine* 2004;29:79–86.
Straus BN. Chronic pain of spinal origin: the costs of intervention. *Spine* 2002;27(22):2614–9.

Randomized Controlled Trial

North RB, Kidd D, Shipley J, et al. Spinal cord stimulation versus reoperation for failed back surgery syndrome: a cost effectiveness and cost utility analysis based on a randomized, controlled trial. *Neurosurgery* 2007;61(2):361–9.

Clinical Trials

Blond S, Buisset N, Dam Hieu P, et al. Cost–benefit evaluation of spinal cord stimulation treatment for failed-back surgery syndrome patients [in French]. *Neurochirurgie* 2004;50(4):443–53.
Kumar K, Malik S, Deneria D. Treatment of chronic pain with spinal cord stimulation versus alternative therapies: cost-effectiveness analysis. *Neurosurgery* 2002;51(1):106–16.
Health Technology Assessment Information Service [a branch of a World Health Organization collaborating center]. *Spinal cord (dorsal column) stimulation for chronic intractable pain,* Plymouth Meeting, PA, ECRI, October 1993.

Modeling Study

Bell GK, Kidd D, North RB. Cost-effectiveness analysis of spinal cord stimulation in treatment of failed back surgery syndrome. *J Pain Symptom Manage* 1997;13:286–95.

Cost Descriptions Lacking Comparators

Bel S, Bauer BL. Dorsal column stimulation (DCS): cost to benefit analysis. *Acta Neurochir* 1991;52(Suppl):121–3.
Budd K. Spinal cord stimulation: cost–benefit study. *Neuromodulation* 2002;5(2):75–8.
Devulder J, de Laat M, van Bastelaere M, et al. Spinal cord stimulation: a valuable treatment for chronic failed back surgery patients. *J Pain Symptom Manage* 1997;13(5):296–301.

Cost-Effectiveness of SCS for CRPS

Randomized Controlled Trial

Kemler MA, Furnee CA. Economic evaluation of spinal cord stimulation for chronic reflex sympathetic dystrophy. *Neurology* 2002; 59:1203–9.

Cost-Effectiveness of SCS for Neuropathic Pain Syndromes

Low Back Pain

Raphael JH, Southall JL, Gnanadurai TV, et al. Chronic mechanical low back pain: a comparative study with intrathecal opioids drug delivery. *Neuromodulation* 2004;7(4):260–6.

Unspecified Indications

Willis KD. A simple approach to outcomes assessment of the therapeutic and cost–benefit success rates for spinal cord stimulation therapy. *Anesthesiol Clin North Am* 2003;21(4):817–23.

Systematic Reviews, Meta-Analyses, and Recommendations

Boswell MV, Trescot AM, Datta S, et al. Interventional techniques: evidence-based practice guidelines in the management of chronic spinal pain. *Pain Phys* 2007;10(7):7–111.

Cameron T. Safety and efficacy of spinal cord stimulation for the treatment of chronic pain: a 20-year literature review. *J Neurosurg Spine* 2004;100(3):254–67.

Carter ML. Spinal cord stimulation in chronic pain: a review of the evidence. *Anaesth Intensive Care* 2004;32(1):11–21.

Grabow TS, Tella PK, Raja SN. Spinal cord stimulation for complex regional pain syndrome: an evidence-based medicine review of the literature. *Clin J Pain* 2003;19(6):371–83.

Henderson JM, Schade CM, Sasaki J, et al. Prevention of mechanical failures in implanted spinal cord stimulation systems. *Neuromodulation* 2006;9(3):183–91.

Kumar K, Buchser E, Linderoth B, et al. Avoiding complications from spinal cord stimulation: practical recommendations from an international panel of experts. *Neuromodulation* 2007;10(1):24–33.

Mailis-Gagnon A, Furlan AD, Sandoval JA, et al. Spinal cord stimulation for chronic pain. *Cochrane Database of Systematic Reviews* 2004; Issue 3. Art. No.: CD003783. DOI: 10.1002/14651858.CD003783.pub2.

Middleton P, Simpson B, Maddern G. Spinal cord stimulation (neurostimulation): an accelerated systematic review. AERSNIP-S R Report No. 43. 2003. Adelaide, South Australia, Australian Safety and Efficacy Register of New Interventional Procedures—Surgical (ASERNIP-S).

Taylor RS. Spinal cord stimulation in complex regional pain syndrome and refractory neuropathic back and leg pain/failed back surgery syndrome: results of a systematic review and meta-analysis. *J Pain Symptom Manage* 2006;31(4 Suppl):S13–9.

Taylor RS, Taylor RJ, Van Buyten J-P, et al. The cost effectiveness of spinal cord stimulation in the treatment of pain: a systematic review of the literature. *J Pain Symptom Manage* 2004;27:370–8.

Taylor RS, Van Buyten J-P, Buchser E. Spinal cord stimulation for complex regional pain syndrome: a systematic review of the clinical and cost-effectiveness literature and assessment of prognostic factors. *Eur J Pain* 2006;10(2):91–101.

Taylor RS, Van Buyten J-P, Buchser E. Spinal cord stimulation for chronic back and leg pain and failed back surgery syndrome: a systematic review and analysis of prognostic factors. *Spine* 2005;30(1):152–60.

Turner JA, Loeser JD, Bell KG. Spinal cord stimulation for chronic low back pain: a systematic literature synthesis. *Neurosurgery* 1995;37:1088–96.

Turner JA, Loeser JD, Deyo RA, et al. Spinal cord stimulation for patients with failed back surgery syndrome or complex regional pain syndrome: a systematic review of effectiveness and complications. *Pain* 2004;108(1):137–47.

Wetzel FT, Hassenbusch S, Oakley JC, et al. Treatment of chronic pain in failed back surgery patients with spinal cord stimulation: a review of current literature and proposal for future investigation. *Neuromodulation* 2000;3(2):59–74.

2

SCS Screening Trial: Patient Selection and Preparation

Introduction

As in any treatment, the success of spinal cord stimulation (SCS) depends on appropriate patient selection. Patients should undergo a thorough evaluation, including a detailed history and physical examination, as well as diagnostic and imaging studies. Conservative measures, including medication trials, interventional procedures, and physical therapy, should be tried unless contraindicated before considering a screening trial of SCS. Patients with appropriate neuropathic pain indications who have failed to respond to initial medication and interventional therapies should be considered for a trial of SCS as early as possible because continually increasing medication dosages often leads to greater disability and side effects. Because certain types of neuropathic pain respond better to SCS than others, the patient's specific pain diagnosis will determine whether or not SCS is indicated and will help the physician assess the likelihood of a successful outcome.

Because SCS is reversible and minimally invasive, a trial of SCS should precede certain irreversible surgical interventions such as sympathectomies or major reconstructive procedures in selected patients with complex regional pain syndrome (CRPS) or previous failed back surgery, respectively. There is some evidence to suggest that SCS may be less successful in patients with more numerous prior interventions and longer duration of pain.[1–5] A trial of SCS has the additional advantage of duplicating the beneficial effects, side effects, and technical interface of the implanted system. Few surgical interventions provide a mode of predicting success or failure prior to fully committing. The screening trial therefore provides patients with the means of determining whether an implanted SCS system will benefit them.

Matching the patient to the physician's own skill set is another important consideration in selecting a patient for SCS. Implanters who do not have the training or experience necessary to be successful should not undertake a complex or difficult procedure. An experienced physician should perform the surgery on patients with challenging anatomy such as obesity, severe spondylosis or scoliosis, or a medical condition that precludes them from comfortably maintaining a prone position. It is also recommended that implanters perform a sufficient number of straightforward lumbar SCS cases so they feel comfortable before implanting an SCS in the cervical region, where both the degree of difficulty and potential for complication are greater.

If the patient's pain diagnosis supports an SCS trial and the required skills and experience are present, a psychological assessment should rule out major psychiatric pathology and substance abuse in order to establish the patient's ability to cope with a foreign object/medical device within his or her body as well as the patient's willingness and ability to operate the equipment and adhere to treatment plans. Finally, it must be determined whether the patient has any medical conditions or anatomic variations that may make a trial technically difficult or even contraindicated.

Patient Selection

Before performing a trial of SCS, a comprehensive history, physical examination, imaging studies, and a psychological evaluation must be obtained to determine whether the patient has a pain indication that is likely to respond to SCS therapy and to rule out contraindications to performing the procedure.

Indications for Spinal Cord Stimulation

The primary purpose of SCS is to reduce the frequency, duration, and intensity of pain.[6,7] Over the past 40 years, research has found SCS to be effective for several causes of pain. As the technology evolves, however, new indications are being investigated. The FDA-approved indications, investigational applications, and the other applications for SCS with lower success rates are provided here and are current as of November 2007. Contraindications, warnings, and adverse events are also identified.

FDA-Approved Indications

The FDA has approved SCS as a tool in managing chronic, intractable pain of the trunk or limbs, including unilateral or bilateral pain associated with failed back surgery syndrome (FBSS), intractable low back pain, and leg pain.

Within these indications, the success of SCS varies depending on the type of pain. A higher probability of success has been associated with the following:

- *FBSS or postlaminectomy pain*: FBSS is an umbrella term that describes persistent or recurrent pain, mainly of the lower back and legs, that remains after unsuccessful spinal surgery. Between 20% and 40% of the 200,000 Americans who have back surgery each year experience FBSS, making it the most common indication for SCS in the United States.[8] When medical management is unsuccessful, SCS in combination with physical therapy and/or spinal injections may be preferable to reoperation.[8]

  Because FBSS is a diagnosis of exclusion, the presence of surgically correctable lesions must be ruled out through evaluation with imaging studies and surgical consultation. Imaging studies may also reveal the presence of epidural or perineural fibrosis or arachnoiditis, which do not respond to surgery but may respond to SCS. Treatment is more likely to be successful in patients presenting with predominately neuropathic leg (radicular) pain who are treated within 3 years of back surgery.[6] FBSS may occur with or without arachnoiditis or lumbar adhesive arachnoiditis.

- *Radiculopathy*: Radiculopathy results from nerve root damage and can produce neurogenic pain. Radiculopathy may be associated with FBSS or a herniated disk. Pain due to radiculitis or radiculopathy often responds well to SCS. However, other causes of referred or radiating pain— such as facet disease, sacroiliac arthropathy, internal disk disruption, piriformis syndrome, and myofascial pain— must first be ruled out or treated before attempting SCS.[8]

- *Plexopathy*: Plexopathy is a form of neuropathy. Within the peripheral nervous system, several plexus are often associated with neuropathy and pain. Plexopathies, such as brachial plexopathy, are often initially diagnosed by a careful evaluation of the patient's history and symptoms, but electromyography and nerve conduction studies are often the most accurate way to determine the nature and site of the plexopathy. Symptoms related to plexopathies can be mild or severe, from diffuse irritation to intense and intractable pain.

- *Arachnoiditis*: Arachnoiditis is a chronic inflammation and scarring of the meninges at the exit site of the nerve roots from the spinal cord that can occur after spine surgery. Arachnoiditis involves inflammation of the arachnoid membrane that covers the spinal cord and brain,

leading to gradual collection of fibrotic scar tissue that tethers the nerves to the arachnoid membrane. This scarring disrupts the flow of cerebrospinal fluid around the nerves and deprives them of nutrition.

- *Epidural fibrosis*: The symptoms of epidural fibrosis appear at 6 to 12 weeks after back surgery and often follow an initial period of pain relief, after which recurrent leg pain may slowly develop.

- *Painful peripheral neuropathy*: More than 100 types of peripheral neuropathy have been identified, each with its own characteristic symptoms, pattern of development, and prognosis. Impaired function and symptoms depend on the type of nerves damaged: motor, sensory, or autonomic.

- *Multiple sclerosis*: In a study published in 2006, 15 of 19 patients with lower extremity pain secondary to multiple sclerosis obtained good pain relief with SCS therapy.[4]

- *CRPS*, type I (formerly called reflex sympathetic dystrophy) or type II (formerly called causalgia): A known nerve injury characterizes CRPS type II but is absent in CRPS type I. CRPS is a syndrome most often caused by trauma and includes burning pain, hyperesthesia, swelling, hyperhidrosis, and trophic changes in the skin and bone of the affected areas. The goal of SCS is to restore function to the affected limb. A trial of SCS should be considered, particularly if patients do not respond to conventional treatment within 16 weeks.[1,4,6,9] Success is associated with a diagnosis of CRPS type I, a limb affected for at least 6 months that does not respond to less invasive therapies, a baseline pain score of at least 5 on a 10-point visual analog scale, and a response of increased mobility to sympathetic blockade.[6]

A reduced probability of success has been associated with the following:[1,4,9]

- Axial spine pain associated with FBSS[10]
- Postherpetic neuralgia
- Post-thoracotomy pain
- Phantom pain
- Intercostal neuralgia
- Incomplete spinal cord injury

In our experience, as well as that of other implanters, many patients with a diagnosis that is not as strongly correlated with a positive outcome have done extremely well with SCS. Numerous case reports of patients with phantom pain, post-thoracotomy pain, partial spinal cord injury, inguinal neuralgia, and post-herniorrhaphy pain[11] have documented lasting pain reduction with SCS. This wide variation in response to SCS is not surprising in the setting of partial spinal cord injury given that each of these neuronal injuries is unique with varying reactions by the host to incomplete cord damage and differences in neuroplastic response. What is more puzzling is the variation in response to SCS among patients with presumed identical pathology, such as phantom limb pain or postherpetic neuralgia. Clearly, this is an area of intense interest to many in the field of neuromodulation.

Off-label Applications

One indication for SCS with strong evidence for a high degree of efficacy is ischemic pain in either peripheral vascular disease or refractory angina.[8,12,13] However, this indication is not currently approved by the FDA. SCS has a profound effect on sympathetic vascular tone and promotes local blood flow and ischemic ulcer healing in patients with peripheral vascular disease.[14]

SCS is most commonly used in Europe for these indications, which is where most of the studies have been conducted. Documented evidence for its efficacy has led to increasing support for use of SCS in the treatment of peripheral vascular disease or refractory angina in the United States. Despite the off-label use for refractory angina, some insurers are now covering SCS for this indication.[15]

Several other pain conditions are being studied for possible applications of SCS. SCS for axial low back pain from mechanical causes has received a great deal of attention but requires more study to determine long-term efficacy. In addition to our experience, other implanters have also noted that axial low back pain from mechanical causes often does not respond well to SCS. Although a significant subset of patients with neuropathic axial back pain may experience long-term improvement with SCS, the success rate is probably lower than that for patients with radiculopathies or CRPS.

An offshoot of SCS is spinal nerve root stimulation. This differs from SCS in that rather than stimulating the dorsal columns of the spinal cord, electrical current is applied directly to one or more spinal nerve roots. Many creative approaches to nerve root stimulation have been described. Leads can be placed in the lumbar epidural space using a retrograde approach (toward the foot) such that lumbar and sacral roots can be stimulated directly. Transforaminal and extraforaminal nerve root stimulation has also been described, allowing specific nerve roots to be targeted. Techniques for performing spinal nerve root stimulation are outside of the scope of this text and are not covered in detail.[16–23]

Another application of stimulation technology—peripheral nerve stimulation—is being studied to treat migraine headaches and other peripheral neuropathies, such as ilioinguinal neuralgia. Efficacy has not yet been established for either of these applications, although large-scale clinical trials are underway. Anecdotal evidence suggests that peripheral nerve stimulation may be an important approach in the future.

Unsuccessful Applications

SCS has been applied to several conditions with unacceptable success rates. These pain syndromes may not be amenable to stimulation because of profound centralization or unidentified areas of the nervous system that currently cannot be stimulated with conventional methods. These conditions include:

- Spinal cord injury with complete cord transection[7]
- Paraplegia and quadriplegia[9]
- Partial spinal cord injury with loss of posterior column function[7]
- Brachial plexus or other nerve root avulsion[9]
- Nonischemic, nociceptive pain[7]
- Central pain of nonspinal origin[7,9]

Contraindications

SCS is not suitable for all patients. Contraindications can be divided into three categories: anatomic conditions, medical comorbidities, and psychosocial considerations.

Relative contraindications to the percutaneous screening trial are:

- Anatomic conditions
  - Previous spinal surgery with epidural scarring in the anticipated path of the SCS leads or severe spondylosis or scoliosis with anticipated difficult entry of the leads into the epidural space (depends on skill and experience of surgeon)
- Medical comorbidities
  - Untreated infection
  - Implanted cardiac pacemaker, cardioverter, or defibrillator. (Note: With improved technology, the presence of a pacemaker may not rule out SCS placement. Technical support services for both pacemaker and stimulator manufacturers should be contacted for final determination.)
  - Existence of a major additional chronic pain condition
  - Anticoagulant or antiplatelet therapy
- Psychosocial considerations
  - Psychological instability or unresolved psychiatric comorbidity
  - Ongoing litigation with the possibility of secondary gain
  - Inconsistencies on history, physical examination (presence of inorganic signs), and diagnostic studies
  - Occupational considerations (e.g., job requires ladder climbing)

Contraindications to SCS therapy are:[24,25]
- Anatomic conditions
  - Pregnancy[25]
  - Previous dorsal root entry zone lesions[24]
  - Critical central spinal stenosis[25]
  - Serious neurologic deficit with surgically correctable pathology[25]
  - Anatomic spine instability at risk for progression[25]
- Medical comorbidities
  - Need for future magnetic resonance imaging (MRI)[25]
  - Coagulopathy, immunosuppression, or other medical condition resulting in unacceptable surgical risk[25]
  - Ongoing requirement for therapeutic diathermy[25]
- Psychosocial considerations
  - Severe cognitive impairment and/or inability to operate the device[25]
  - Unacceptable living situation or social environment[25]
  - Active substance abuse[25]

Anatomic Considerations

Epidural Access and Stenosis

A trial of SCS depends on the ability to successfully place the stimulator leads within the epidural space. In patients with low back or leg pain, the leads will usually be inserted at an intervertebral space somewhere between T12 and L3 and directed anterograde (toward the head) in the thoracic epidural space. In patients with upper extremity pain, the leads will usually be inserted within the intervertebral space somewhere between T2 and T6 and directed anterograde in the cervical epidural space.

Spine Abnormalities

In all cases, the portion of the spine through which the leads will pass must be accessible, with sufficient space to accommodate a lead. Several abnormalities of the spine are common in candidates for SCS and must be considered before proceeding with a trial.

Spondylosis

Osteophytes that accompany severe spondylosis may make identification of and access to the intralaminar space more difficult. This is especially true at the thoracic level because of the relatively reduced size of the thoracic intralaminar space. Hypertrophy of the ligamentum flavum can make a routine procedure more difficult. Plain x-rays can be helpful in identifying bony abnormalities such as osteophytes at the intralaminar space so that a preoperative approach can be planned. Having those films available for reference in the operating room at the time of surgery can also be helpful. Unfortunately, it is not always possible to predict which patients are going to be challenging, even when radiographs and imaging studies are immediately available.

Previous Back Surgery

Previous back surgeries resulting in epidural scarring, spinal fusion, the presence of lumbar or cervical stenosis, or severe anatomic variations such as scoliosis or kyphosis, can make access difficult and even dangerous. Multiple back surgeries can result in epidural scarring that extends beyond the surgical level. The presence of epidural scarring can affect loss of resistance with the Tuohy needle and make attempts to pass an epidural lead hazardous.

Spinal Stenosis

Spinal stenosis and other epidural pathologies can be diagnosed only on imaging studies. Central canal stenosis, if present, is typically diagnosed by radiologists after reviewing sagittal MRI images.[26] The diagnosis must be ruled out because subclinical stenosis may result in frank myelopathy when a space-occupying lead is placed into the epidural space. In the cervical spine, the mid-sagittal diameter is used to diagnose stenosis. An anterior–posterior (AP) diameter of less than 14 mm is cause for concern and, if possible, a neuroradiologist

should be consulted before proceeding with a trial. An AP diameter of less than 10 mm in the cervical spine is a contraindication to the placement of a percutaneous epidural stimulator lead.[26]

In any event, if the radiology report notes central canal stenosis, the images should be reviewed, preferably with a neuroradiologist, to determine whether the epidural space can accommodate stimulator leads.[26]

Medical Considerations

Coagulopathy

Managing the anticoagulated patient about to undergo a neuraxial procedure has become more challenging and complex. An epidural hematoma following a procedure involving the neuraxis remains a major concern. Medical standards for preventing venous thromboembolism are being widely implemented. Additionally, more efficacious anticoagulants and antiplatelet agents are available, and new ones are being developed. Although epidural hematoma is rare (one review estimated the incidence to be 0.0006%),[27] the devastating consequences associated with this complication, including possible permanent paralysis, make it an important risk factor requiring serious consideration.

The American Society of Regional Anesthesia and Pain Medicine (ASRA) published consensus guidelines in 2003 for the use of neuraxial anesthesia and analgesia in patients receiving anticoagulants. The ASRA guidelines note that numerous studies have documented the safety of neuraxial anesthesia and analgesia in these patients, which is predicated on "appropriate timing of needle placement and catheter removal relative to the timing of anticoagulant drug administration."[28]

Even if we assume that placing an SCS lead is analogous to placing an epidural infusion catheter, and that the lead can be safely placed, there are no data on the long-term risk of epidural hematoma in patients with indwelling epidural SCS leads who have been anticoagulated or who have a genetic or acquired coagulopathy. Some neurosurgeons believe that a paddle lead, which is less likely to move, may be safer than a percutaneous lead in a patient requiring long-term anticoagulation. Other implanters believe that paddle leads increase the risk of bleeding as a result of laminotomy and the extent of surgery required to place these leads. Both positions are speculative.

The issue of anticoagulation is important in Europe because SCS is often used to treat refractory angina, and cardiac patients are often anticoagulated for various reasons. Such patients can be stratified into risk categories for purposes of SCS. Low-risk patients are those with atrial fibrillation and no history of embolic events, whereas high-risk patients are those with prosthetic valve replacements.[29]

The National Refractory Angina Centre in Liverpool has published guidelines for SCS placement in low- and high-risk cardiac patients requiring anticoagulation.[29] The authors note that there is currently no evidence of increased risk of epidural hematoma in patients with stable leads in the epidural space. However, with a rare event, many people need to be studied in order to make that claim. The National Refractory Angina Centre also notes that SCS is the "most promising therapeutic option" for many of their cardiac patients, and for that reason, there is no risk-free option. However, a lack of data does not imply a lack of risk, so caution and conservative management are recommended when treating patients taking anticoagulants or platelet inhibitors.

All patients should be evaluated for hemostasis and coagulation disorders. An accurate history and physical provide the most valuable information for assessing the risk of bleeding.[30] In particular, one should look for a personal or family history of the following:

- Easy bruising (spontaneous or traumatic)
- Frequent or unusual mucosal bleeding
- Irregular, prolonged, and excessive menstrual flow
- Hematuria
- Epistaxis
- Marked or life-threatening hemorrhage with invasive procedures
- Liver dysfunction
- Renal dysfunction
- Major metabolic or endocrine disorders

Patients should always be asked about the medications they are taking. In particular, they should be questioned specifically about aspirin and nonsteroidal anti-inflammatory drug use because they often do not consider these medications important enough to mention without prompting.

Several screening tests are available for bleeding disorders. However, in otherwise normal patients, these tests do not add appreciably to what can be learned from a good history and physical examination.

Infection

All patients should be evaluated for active infection. Systemic infections, such as pneumonia, bronchitis, or urinary tract infections, must be treated and resolved before the patient undergoes a trial of SCS or permanent implantation. A local infection or inflammatory process, such as psoriasis or other rashes, at the implant site also should be resolved before a trial.

Suppressed Immune Response

Patients with renal disease, diabetes, cancer in remission, or chronic illness may have a suppressed immune response, putting them at increased risk for infection with SCS. Patients with poor nutritional status such as malabsorption secondary to gastric bypass or other chronic illnesses such as rheumatoid arthritis, lupus, or HIV also have compromised immune systems that increase the risk with SCS. Individuals with diabetes and peripheral neuropathy will often respond well to SCS; however, they should be under optimal glycemic control

before proceeding with a trial. Patients with any chronic illness should be medically and nutritionally optimized to the greatest extent possible. Many of these patients can benefit greatly from SCS with increased levels of functioning that can lead to improvement in their chronic illness. For instance, many of our patients with diabetes have been able to engage more actively in exercise and other activities once their peripheral neuropathy is under better control.

Recently, there has been increased interest in neuromodulation therapy for cancer survivors with chronic pain. With ongoing advances in chemotherapy, radiation, and surgery, many patients with cancer are living longer. Unfortunately, many are left with iatrogenic neuropathic pain from chemotherapy, surgery, and radiation. With the advent of improved SCS systems, many patients with cancer and post-thoracotomy pain can be optimally treated with a combination of medications and SCS. Currently, patients with cancer who require ongoing monitoring with MRI are not candidates for SCS implantation.

Our philosophy is to medically optimize our patients while weighing the risks and benefits before proceeding. Fortunately, SCS implantation results in relatively minimal physiologic stress, especially compared with other more invasive surgeries.

Tobacco Abuse

In our general pain practice, we find that a high percentage of pain patients smoke. These patients are at increased risk for infection and other surgical complications if they have surgery, including SCS. Because of this increased risk, many surgeons will not perform elective surgery on smokers.

Rates of wound infection are significantly higher in smokers than in nonsmokers. Patients who smoke and have joint replacement surgery, breast reconstruction, facelifts, and a variety of other plastic surgery procedures have up to an eightfold[31] increase in wound infections and wound dehiscence compared with nonsmokers. In a study of patients undergoing breast reconstruction, abdominal wall site necrosis occurred in 7.9% of current smokers compared with 1% of nonsmokers. Mastectomy-flap necrosis occurred in 7.7% of smokers compared with 1.5% of nonsmokers. In patients having abdominoplasty, wound dehiscence requiring repeat surgery was seen in 24% of smokers but only 8.2% of nonsmokers.[31] Smoking cessation was examined in a randomized study in patients undergoing joint replacement surgery. In patients who quit smoking, wound infection rates were reduced from 27% to 0%. It appears that simply reducing the amount smoked does not decrease the risk. The optimal period of smoking cessation is probably at least 6 weeks.[32] In one study, termination of smoking for less than 3 weeks before colorectal surgery was not associated with a reduction in risk.

Although the absolute cause for the increased wound infection rate is not definite, there are more than 3,000 chemical byproducts associated with smoking, of which nicotine is the most studied.[31] Carbon monoxide levels in smokers decrease tissue oxygenation sufficiently to result in clinically significant hypoxia, which has been shown to impair wound healing in animals.[31]

The benefits of smoking cessation appear at about 4 weeks and continue for the next 4 weeks. It takes 1 to 2 months to start reversing the effects of small airway disease and to clear secretions. Studies show that patients who are able to quit for more than 4 to 6 weeks may reduce their rate of postoperative complications by 50%.[32] Our policy is based on literature showing evidence that patients who quit smoking for 6 weeks or more have a risk reduction almost to that of nonsmokers. Because SCS is an elective intervention and an expensive resource that focuses on improving function, we have a firm no-smoking policy for at least 6 weeks before the trial. For some patients, this may be the incentive they need to quit for good.[33–35]

Establishing Medical Necessity

A statement of medical necessity may need to be provided to payers when recommending SCS for patients in chronic pain. The implanter must certify that the patient meets the indications for SCS, that previous therapies have not been successful, and that SCS offers a reasonable chance of success (see Appendix A).

Psychosocial Considerations

Pain is experienced not only as a consequence of the neuroplastic changes that occur after an injury, but also within the context of the patient's medical history. Pain at the most basic level is experienced as a threat to the individual. Therefore, patients in pain respond in an attempt to reduce and eliminate this dysphoric sensation. Unsuccessful attempts to alleviate pain can result in coping difficulties, which may in turn result in anxiety, frustration, anger, and depression. Unrelenting pain is known to produce neuroplastic changes in the spinal cord and brain leading to changes in neurotransmitter concentrations and neural connections. These hardwiring changes often result in alterations of mood, motivation, and affect. Patients in chronic pain may have difficulty differentiating their pain from other psychological symptoms, which may result in a tendency to amplify pain symptoms. Patients may also have trouble adopting recommended behavior changes because of a sense of hopelessness and powerlessness. The degree and impact of psychological symptoms vary significantly from person to person, but they should be assessed and treated whenever possible.

Severe pain is often accompanied by affective disturbances such as depression and anxiety. In fact, most patients with chronic pain have a mixture of depression, hypochondriasis, and anxiety or emotional reactivity.[36] Thus, a psychosocial evaluation is a necessary part of an interdisciplinary approach to treating chronic pain.[37] Psychological factors may be mediators, modulators, or maintainers of pain[38] and should be assessed with this fact in mind.

Psychological Contraindications and Testing

Although many patients with pain also suffer from depression and anxiety, it is the role that these affective states play in the patient's experience of pain that is important in determining whether the patient is a candidate for SCS. Some patients have preexisting psychiatric disorders that become magnified by pain. Some implanters may consider several of the following psychiatric diagnoses to be contraindications for SCS:[36,39]

- Personality disorders
- Unstable or unsupportive family and personal relationships
- Suicidal tendencies
- Severe depression or mood disorder
- Severe sleep disturbances
- Somatization or somatoform disorder
- Active alcohol or drug abuse
- Marked cognitive deficits that prevent the patient from properly operating the system. Cognitive impairment, by itself, is not a contraindication; however, the patient must have a competent caregiver and adequate social support in this instance.

Although psychological testing does not predict outcome, it can be used to identify comorbid psychiatric conditions and psychological factors that should be addressed before SCS is considered. Testing may suggest treatments for psychological risk factors and specific pain syndromes and determine the patient's personal ability and available support systems for coping with pain.[6,7,38] Psychological testing can also establish a baseline against which post-implant improvement can be assessed.[7] Certain insurance carriers, such as workers' compensation carriers, may require a psychological evaluation before giving authorization for the procedure.

The following tests are frequently used to assess a patient's suitability for a trial of SCS:

- To evaluate pain intensity: McGill Pain Questionnaire, numeric rating scales, visual analog scales, verbal rating scales, and pain drawings
- To evaluate mood and personality and overall psychological functioning: Minnesota Multiphasic Personality Inventory-2, Symptom Checklist 90-R, Beck Depression Inventory, Spielberger State-Trait Anxiety Inventory, Millon Behavior Health Inventory, Illness Behavior Questionnaire, Pain Assessment Inventory, Derogatis Affects Balance Scale, Roland Morris Questionnaire, Hospital Anxiety and Depression Scale, and Perceived Stress Scale
- To assess pain beliefs and coping: Multidimensional Pain Inventory, Chronic Illness Problem Inventory, Coping Strategies Questionnaire, Pain Management Inventory, Pain Self-Efficacy Questionnaire, Survey of Pain Attitudes, Sickness Impact Profile, Inventory of Negative Thoughts in Response to Pain, Pain Beliefs Inventory, and Pain Locus of Control Scale

- To assess level of functioning: Multidimensional Pain Inventory, Oswestry Disability Questionnaire, Sickness Impact Profile, Short-Form Health Survey, Social Support Questionnaire, and Pain Disability Index
- To evaluate cognitive functioning: Mini-Mental State.

Psychological contraindications to SCS are cited in the contraindications section.

Characteristics that, in our experience and the experience of others, are associated with positive SCS outcomes include the following:[36]

- General psychological stability
- Adequate self-confidence and self-efficacy
- Realistic assessment of the medical problem and expectations of treatment
- General optimism regarding outcome
- Ability to cope with side effects, complications, and flare-ups without catastrophizing
- Adequate training in operating the pulse generator
- A supportive and educated family
- Willingness to undergo comprehensive medical and lifestyle evaluations[37]

Many patients with pain view psychological assessment with deep suspicion, especially if they are involved in litigation. When recommending a psychological assessment, patients may accept the term "behavioral pain assessment" more readily than "psychiatric" or "mental health" evaluation.

Patient Education

Evidence strongly supports the benefits of informing patients about the procedural and experiential aspects of stimulator and lead implantation before the trial.[38] In particular, patients should have realistic expectations about the technology, including the chances for failure. They need to know that complete pain relief is unlikely but that partial pain relief is probable.[37] Outcomes may be influenced in part by the patient's expectations.

Knowing the patient's priorities may help focus educational and counseling efforts. The secret is to balance hope against unrealistic expectations. Surgical complications are most affected by surgical skill and stimulator characteristics. Pain relief is most affected by the patient's psychological and physiologic state. Patient satisfaction is most affected by the patient's expectations and perceptions of the surgeon, technology, and perioperative experience. Quality of life is most affected by changes in functional and psychological status.[36]

Psychological Preparation

Each patient undergoing an SCS trial has a unique set of feelings, expectations, beliefs, personality traits, dysfunctions, experiences, support systems, and skills. Fully preparing patients for the procedure can reduce their anxiety, improve their adherence to recommendations, and optimize outcomes

as well as reduce unnecessary post-implant office visits and phone calls. Frequently asked questions are outlined in Appendix B.

Considerable research has established that greater distress or anxiety before surgery is associated with greater postoperative pain and a slower and more complicated recovery.[37,38] Presurgical psychosocial interventions generally have positive effects on postsurgical physical and psychological functioning, as well as leading to faster and stronger recovery, shorter hospital stays, fewer postoperative complications, better adherence to treatment recommendations, less use of analgesics, and improved measures of cardiovascular and respiratory functions.[38]

Patients often want to talk with others who already have implanted SCS systems.[37] Many have questions about recharging batteries, changes in daily activities, concern with the appearance of the subcutaneous stimulator, apprehension about having a foreign object permanently implanted in their spine, and so on. Uncontrolled postoperative pain is also a common fear. Talking with others can be a valuable experience for surgical candidates, although the individual differences in the efficacy of SCS should be emphasized to avoid the appearance of endorsing the technology.[37]

Presurgical instruction in relaxation methods and stress management can be effective in reducing pain and accelerating healing.[37] Chronic insomnia and nonrestorative sleep are common in patients with severe pain, so information about improving sleep and the use of medications to improve sleep can be helpful.

Many patients are concerned that increasing their activity levels after implantation will increase their pain or cause nerve damage. Such anticipatory anxiety may result in reduced activity or prompt the recurrence of severe pain. It is well known that patients' attitudes and beliefs about their pain influence the efficacy of any pain treatment that is undertaken.

Negative treatment outcomes are more likely when patients believe the following:

- Pain is purely a physical problem that can be resolved only with the right treatment.[38]
- Psychosocial factors play little or no role in pain or pain treatment.[38]
- Chronic pain means the loss of a normal life.[39,40]
- I cannot have an impact on my own pain.[41–43]
- I will not get better.[39,40,43]

Negative outcomes are also more likely when patients behave as passive bystanders in the treatment process and have significant others who enable "sick" behaviors and undermine "well" behaviors.

Positive treatment outcomes are more likely with the following patient beliefs:

- Pain has multiple components and is best treated with a multidimensional approach.[42,43]
- The benefits of pain control outweigh the risks.[41]
- I can affect treatment outcomes.[42,43]

- I can learn and adopt coping skills—and techniques for applying the skills—to manage the self-defeating beliefs and behaviors that contribute to pain.[39]
- I can be an active partner on the treatment team.[39,41]

Positive outcomes are more likely when patients have significant others who reinforce positive behavioral changes and do not expect treatment to relieve all their pain all the time.[38–43]

Procedural Information

Well in advance of the trial, patients should be told, both in person and in writing, about the efficacy of SCS for their specific indication, as well as about the potential limitations, risks, complications, and adverse effects of the procedure. They should be given at least a general overview of the surgical procedure. Also, it should be emphasized that SCS is but one aspect of their overall pain management program and that the need for care will be ongoing. Patients also need to know how the pulse generator works—how to turn it on and off and how to adjust the rate and amplitude of stimulation. Appendix C is a checklist of the topics that should be covered. Ideally, patients should be exposed to this information several times and through several different media so they understand what to expect. Uncertainty is associated with anxiety, so every effort should be made to address patients' questions and concerns before a trial of SCS.

Patients should limit their activity for 10 to 12 hours after the procedure because bed rest reduces the risk of lead movement. The day after surgery, they may walk for brief periods, keeping their backs as straight as possible to avoid moving the leads.

For the duration of the trial, patients **should not**:

- Raise their arms over their heads or move their shoulders beyond 90 degrees of flexion or abduction
- Bend, twist, stretch, or lift more than 5 lb
- Drive or operate machinery when the stimulator is on, because unexpected electrical surges can cause distracting sensations and unwanted muscle contractions
- Shower or bathe

For the duration of the trial, patients **should**:

- Position their beds to maintain body alignment
- Sleep on a firm mattress that supports their legs and back equally
- Maintain a dry trial lead insertion site by limiting bathing to sponge baths
- Resume sexual activity, unless advised otherwise
- Obtain physician approval before undergoing spinal or chiropractic manipulation
- Move their shoulders and hips at the same time in a "log-rolling" movement that does not twist the spine

Patients should also be informed that, during the trial period, they may experience changes in stimulation when making abrupt movements or shifting position. These changes are caused by the shifting of the lead during movement, and they diminish as scar tissue forms and stabilizes the lead. The following instructions can be helpful:

- If stimulation increases when you bend your neck back or lean back or when you lie down or sit, decrease the stimulation by lowering the amplitude.
- If stimulation decreases when you stand up, increase the stimulation by increasing the amplitude.
- Stimulation may stop when you bend your neck forward or lean forward. Stimulation will resume when you assume a different position. If this occurs too quickly when you move, try increasing the amplitude slightly.
- To smooth out the sensation, adjust the rate of stimulation until you feel comfortable.
- Turn the neurostimulator off or the amplitude down when changing positions or making adjustments.
- If the stimulation is uncomfortable at any time, turn the neurostimulator off.

Informed Consent

Both the trial and permanent implantation of SCS are invasive procedures that carry surgical risk. Written informed consent from the patient is required, but no special circumstances need be added to the standard consent form.

The risks and complications associated with SCS are low compared with other surgical procedures on the spine, but the following risks should be reviewed with the patient:

- Bleeding
- Severe infection or meningitis
- Allergic reactions to anesthetics
- Spinal cord injury or paralysis
- Nerve damage causing numbness or weakness
- Constant pain around the implant site
- Postsurgical soreness
- Possible reduced efficacy of SCS over time
- Battery failure or leakage
- Equipment malfunction
- Lead fracture or migration, resulting in loss of stimulation or electrical shock sensations

REFERENCES

1. Kumar K, Toth C, Nath RK, et al. Epidural spinal cord stimulation for treatment of chronic pain—some predictors of success. A 15-year experience. *Surg Neurol* 1998;50(2):110–20.
2. North RB, Kidd DH, Zahurak M, et al. Spinal cord stimulation for chronic, intractable pain: experience over two decades. *Neurosurgery* 1993;32(3):384–95.
3. North RB, Kidd DH, Farrokhi F, et al. Spinal cord stimulation versus repeated lumbosacral spine surgery for chronic pain: a randomized, controlled trial. *Neurosurgery* 2005;56(1):98–106.
4. Kumar K, Hunter G, Demeria D. Spinal cord stimulation in treatment of chronic benign pain: challenges in treatment planning

and present status, a 22-year experience. *Neurosurgery* 2006; 58(3):481–96.

5. Kumar K, Toth C. The role of spinal cord stimulation in the treatment of chronic pain postlaminectomy. *Curr Pain Headache Rep* 1998;2:85–92.

6. Lee AW, Pilitsis JG. Spinal cord stimulation: indications and outcomes. *Neurosurg Focus* 2006;21:E3.

7. British Pain Society. *Spinal cord stimulation for the management of pain: recommendations for best clinical practice.* London: British Pain Society, 2005.

8. Augustinsson LE. Spinal cord electrical stimulation in severe angina pectoris: surgical technique, intraoperative physiology, complications and side effects. *Pacing Clin Electrophysiol* 1989; 12(4):693–4.

9. Simpson A, Myerson BA, Linderoth B. Spinal cord and brain stimulation. In: McMahon SB, Koltzenburg M, eds. *Wall and Melzack's textbook of pain,* 5th ed. Philadelphia: Elsevier Churchill Livingstone; 2006:569.

10. Fogel GR, Esses SI, Calvillo O. Management of chronic limb pain with spinal cord stimulation. *Pain Pract* 2003;3:144–51.

11. Elias M. Spinal cord stimulation for post-herniorrhaphy pain. *Neuromodulation* 2000;3:155–7.

12. Augustinsson LE. Spinal cord stimulation in peripheral vascular disease and angina pectoris. *J Neurosurg Sci* 2003;47:37–40.

13. Jacobs MJ, Jörning PJ, Joshi SR, et al. Epidural spinal cord electrical stimulation improves microvascular blood flow in severe limb ischemia. *Ann Surg* 1998;207:179–83.

14. Sagher O, Huang D-L. Mechanisms of spinal cord stimulation in ischemia. *Neurosurg Focus* 2006;21(6):1–5.

15. Cigna HealthCare Coverage Position. Spinal cord stimulation: coverage position number: 0380. Cigna Health Corporation, 2007.

16. Haque R, Winfree CJ. Spinal nerve root stimulation. *Neurosurg Focus* 2006;21(6):1–7.

17. Aló KM, Yland MJ, Redko V, et al. Lumbar and sacral nerve root stimulation (NRS) in the treatment of chronic pain: a novel anatomic approach and neurostimulation technique. *Neuromodulation* 1999;2(1):23–31.

18. Dijkema HE, Weil EHJ, Mijs PT, et al. Neuromodulation of sacral nerves for incontinence and voiding dysfunctions. *Eur Urol* 1993;24:72–6.

19. Feler C, Whitworth T, Brookof D, et al. Sacral nerve root stimulation for the treatment of intractable pain due to interstitial cystitis. *Abstracts of American Pain Society Meeting,* 1998.

20. Aló KM, Yland MJ, Redko V. Retrograde intraspinal peripheral neurostimulation: a novel anatomic approach. Proceedings of the International Neuromodulation Society, Number 87. Lucerne, Switzerland, September 1998.

21. Aló KM, Yland MJ, Redko V. Selective lumbar and sacral nerve root stimulation in the treatment of chronic pain. Proceedings of the International Neuromodulation Society, Number 89. Lucerne, Switzerland, September 1998.

22. Aló KM, Feler CA, Oakley J, et al. An in vitro study of electrode placement at the cervical nerve roots using a trans-spinal approach. Proceedings of the International Neuromodulation Society, Number 90. Lucerne, Switzerland, September 1998.

23. Barolat G. Epidural spinal cord stimulation: anatomical and electrical properties of the intraspinal structures relevant to spinal cord stimulation and clinical correlations. *Neuromodulation* 1998;1:63–71.

24. North RB, Wetzel FT. Spinal cord stimulation for chronic pain of spinal origin: a valuable long-term solution. *Spine* 2002;27: 2584–92.

25. North R, Shipley J, Prager J, et al. Practice parameters for the use of spinal cord stimulation in the treatment of chronic neuropathic pain. *Pain Med* 2007;8(4):S200–75.

26. Chapter 102, Imaging Section, in *Grainger and Allison's diagnostic radiology: a textbook of medical imaging,* 4th ed. Churchill Livingstone, 2001.

27. Moraca RJ, Sheldon DG, Thirby RC. The role of epidural anesthesia and analgesia in surgical practice. *Ann Surg* 2003;238: 663–73.

28. Horlocker TT, Wedel DJ, Benzon H, et al. Regional anesthesia in the anticoagulated patient: defining the risks (the second ASRA Consensus Conference on Neuraxial Anesthesia and Anticoagulation). *Reg Anesth Pain Med* 2003;28(3):172–97.

29. Chester MD. Spinal cord stimulation for the treatment of refractory angina. In: UK NHS National Refractory Angina Centre. *Chronic Refractory Angina.* www.angina.org; 2004.

30. Townsend CM, Beauchamp RD, Evers BM, et al. *Sabiston textbook of surgery: the biological basis of modern surgical practice,* 17th ed. Philadelphia: Elsevier, 2004.

31. Peters MJ, Morgan LC, Gluch L. Smoking cessation and elective surgery: the cleanest cut. *Med J Australia* 2004;180(7):317–8.

32. Møller A, Villebro N, Pedersen T, et al. Effect of preoperative smoking intervention on postoperative complications: a randomized clinical trial. *Lancet* 2002;359:114–7.

33. Spear SL, Ducic I, Cuoco F, et al. The effect of smoking on flap and donor-site complications in pedicled TRAM breast reconstruction. *Plastic Reconst Surg* 2005;116:1873–80.

34. Cheadle WG. Risk factors for surgical site infection. *Surg Infect* 2006;7:S7–S11.

35. Neumayer L, Hosokawa P, Itani K, et al. Multivariable predictors of postoperative surgical site infection after general and vascular surgery: results from the Patient Safety in Surgery study. *J Am Coll Surg* 2007;204:1178–87.

36. Doleys D. Psychological factors in spinal cord stimulation therapy: brief review and discussion. *Neurosurg Focus* 2006;21: 1–6.

37. Van Dorsten B. Psychological considerations in preparing patients for implantation procedures. *Pain Med* 2006;7 Suppl 1:S47–S57.

38. Allcock N, Elkan R, Williams J. Patients referred to a pain management clinic: beliefs, expectations and priorities. *J Adv Nurs* 2007;30:248–56.

39. Weisberg MB, Clavel AL. Why is chronic pain so difficult to treat? *Postgrad Med* 1999;106:1–16.

40. Carlsson AM. Personality characteristics of patients with chronic pain in comparison with normal controls and depressed patients. *Pain* 1986;25(3):373–82.

41. Jensen MP, Nielson WR, Kerns RD. Toward the development of a motivational model of pain self-management. *J Pain* 2003;9: 477–92.

42. Coughlin AM, Badura AS, Fleischer TD, et al. Multidisciplinary treatment of chronic pain patients: its efficacy in changing patient locus of control. *Arch Phys Med Rehabil* 2000;8:739–40.

43. Moss-Morris R, Humphrey K, Johnson MH, et al. Patients' perceptions of their pain condition across a multidisciplinary pain management program: do they change and if so does it matter? *Clin J Pain* 2007;23(7):558–64.

Further Reading

FBSS Randomized Controlled Trial

North RB, Kidd DH, Farrokhi F, et al. Spinal cord stimulation versus repeated lumbosacral spine surgery for chronic pain: a randomized, controlled trial. *Neurosurgery* 2005;56(1):98–106.

FBSS Long-Term (at least 24 months) Follow-Up Studies

Blond S, Armignies P, Parker F, et al. Chronic sciatalgia caused by sensitive deafferentiation following surgery for lumbar disk hernia: clinical and therapeutic aspects. Apropos of 110 patients [in French]. *Neurochirurgie* 1991;37(2):86–95.

Budd K. Spinal cord stimulation: cost–benefit study. *Neuromodulation* 2002;5(2):75–8.

Dario A, Fortini G, Bertollo D, et al. Treatment of failed back surgery syndrome. *Neuromodulation* 2001;4(3):105–10.

De Andres J, Quiroz C, Villanueva V, et al. Patient satisfaction with spinal cord stimulation for failed back surgery syndrome [in Spanish]. *Rev Esp Anestesiol Reanim* 2007;54(1):17–22.

de la Porte C, Siegfried J. Lumbosacral spinal fibrosis (spinal arachnoiditis). Its diagnosis and treatment by spinal cord stimulation. *Spine* 1983;8(6):593–603.

de la Porte C, Van de Kelft E. Spinal cord stimulation in failed back surgery syndrome. *Pain* 1993;52(1):55–61.

Devulder J, de Laat M, van Bastelaere M, et al. Spinal cord stimulation: a valuable treatment for chronic failed back surgery patients. *J Pain Symptom Manage* 1997;13(5):296–301.

Fiume D, Sherkat S, Callovini GM, et al. Treatment of the failed back surgery syndrome due to lumbo-sacral epidural fibrosis. *Acta Neurochir Suppl* 1995;64:116–8.

Kumar K, Malik S, Demeria D. Treatment of chronic pain with spinal cord stimulation versus alternative therapies: cost-effectiveness analysis. *Neurosurgery* 2002;51(1):106–15.

Kumar K, Toth C. The role of spinal cord stimulation in the treatment of chronic pain postlaminectomy. *Curr Pain Headache Rep* 1998;2:85–92.

Leclercq TA, Russo E. Epidural stimulation for pain control [in French]. *Neurochirurgie* 1981;27(2):125–8.

North RB, Ewend MG, Lawton MT, et al. Failed back surgery syndrome: 5-year follow-up after spinal cord stimulator implantation. *Neurosurgery* 1991;28(5):692–9.

North RB, Kidd DH, Olin J, et al. Spinal cord stimulation for axial low back pain: a prospective, controlled trial comparing dual with single percutaneous electrodes. *Spine* 2005;30(12):1412–8.

North RB, Kidd DH, Petrucci L, et al. Spinal cord stimulation electrode design: a prospective, randomized, controlled trial comparing percutaneous with laminectomy electrodes: Part II, clinical outcomes. *Neurosurgery* 2005;57(5):990–5.

Probst C. Spinal cord stimulation in 112 patients with epi-/intradural fibrosis following operation for lumbar disc herniation. *Acta Neurochir (Wien)* 1990;107(3-4):147–51.

Rainov NG, Heidecke V, Burkert W. Short test-period spinal cord stimulation for failed back surgery syndrome. *Minim Invasive Neurosurg* 1996;39(2):41–4.

van Buyten J-P, van Zundert JV, Milbouw G. Treatment of failed back surgery syndrome patients with low back and leg pain: a pilot study of a new dual lead spinal cord stimulation system. *Neuromodulation* 1999;2(3):258–65.

FBSS Short-Term Follow-Up Studies

Batier C, Frerebeau P, Kong A, et al. Posterior spinal cord neurostimulation in lumbar radiculitis pain. Apropos of 14 cases [in French]. *Agressologie* 1989;30(3):137–8.

Bel S, Bauer BL. Dorsal column stimulation (DCS): cost to benefit analysis. *Acta Neurochir* 1991;52(suppl):121–3.

De Mulder PA, te Rijdt B, Veeckmans G, et al. Evaluation of a dual quadripolar surgically implanted spinal cord stimulation lead for failed back surgery patients with chronic low back and leg pain. *Neuromodulation* 2005;8(4):219–24.

Fassio B, Sportes J, Romain M, et al. Chronic medullary neuro-stimulation in lumbosacral spinal arachnoiditis [in French]. *Rev Chir Orthop Reparatrice Appar Mot* 1988;74(5):473–9.

Heidecke V, Rainov NG, Burkert W. Hardware failures in spinal cord stimulation for failed back surgery syndrome. *Neuromodulation* 2000;3(1):27–30.

Leclercq TA, Russo E. Epidural stimulation for pain control [in French]. *Neurochirurgie* 1981;27(2):125–8.

LeDoux MS, Langford KH. Spinal cord stimulation for the failed back syndrome. *Spine* 1993;18(2):191–4.

Leveque JC, Villavicencio AT, Bulsara KR, et al. Spinal cord stimulation for failed back surgery syndrome. *Neuromodulation* 2001;4(1):1–9.

North RB, Kidd DH, Olin J, et al. Spinal cord stimulation for axial low back pain: a prospective, controlled trial comparing 16-contact insulated electrode arrays with 4-contact percutaneous electrodes. *Neuromodulation* 2006;9(1):56–67.

Ohnmeiss DD, Rashbaum RF, Bogdanffy GM. Prospective outcome evaluation of spinal cord stimulation in patients with intractable leg pain. *Spine* 1996;21(11):1344–50.

Rutten S, Komp M, Godolias G. Spinal cord stimulation (SCS) using an 8-pole electrode and double-electrode system as minimally invasive therapy of the post-discotomy and post-fusion syndrome—prospective study results in 34 patients [in German]. *Z Orthop Ihre Grenzgeb* 2002;140(6):626–31.

Sharan A, Cameron T, Barolat G. Evolving patterns of spinal cord stimulation in patients implanted for intractable low back and leg pain. *Neuromodulation* 2002;5(3):167–79.

FBSS Case Studies

Arxer A, Busquets C, Vilaplana J, et al. Subacute epidural abscess after spinal cord stimulation implantation. *Eur J Anesthesiol* 2003;20:753–9.

Buonocore M, Demartini L, Bonezzi C. Lumbar spinal cord stimulation can improve muscle strength and gait independently of the analgesic effect: a case report. *Neuromodulation* 2006;9(4):309–13.

FBSS Miscellaneous Studies

North RB, Lanning A, Hessels R, et al. Spinal cord stimulation with percutaneous and plate electrodes: side effects and quantitative comparisons. *Neurosurg Focus* 1997;2(1:3):1–5.

Vijayan R, Ahmad TS. Spinal cord stimulation for treatment of failed back surgery syndrome—two case reports. *Med J Malaysia* 1999;54(4):509–13.

FBSS in Studies With Mixed Indications

Abejón D, Reig E, del Pozo C, et al. Dual spinal cord stimulation for complex pain: preliminary study. *Neuromodulation* 2005;8(2):105–11.

Allegri M, Arachi G, Barbieri M, et al. Prospective study of the success and efficacy of spinal cord stimulation. *Minerva Anestesiol* 2004;70(3):117–24.

Aló KM, Redko V, Charnov J. Four year follow-up of dual electrode spinal cord stimulation for chronic pain. *Neuromodulation* 2002;5(2):79–99.

Aló KM, Yland MJ, Charnov JH, et al. Multiple program spinal cord stimulation in the treatment of chronic pain: follow-up of multiple program SCS. *Neuromodulation* 1999;2(4):266–72.

Aló KM, Yland MJ, Charnov J, et al. Computer-assisted and patient interactive programming of dual electrode spinal cord stimulation in the treatment of chronic pain. *Neuromodulation* 1998;1:1.

Aló KM. Spinal cord stimulation for complex pain: initial experience with a dual electrode, programmable, internal pulse generator. *Pain Practice* 2003;3(1):31–8.

Aló KM, Holsheimer J. New trends in neuromodulation for the management of neuropathic pain. *Neurosurgery* 2002;50(4):690–704.

Broggi G, Servello D, Dones I, et al. Italian multicentric study on pain treatment with epidural spinal cord stimulation. *Stereotact Funct Neurosurg* 1994;62(1–4):273–8.

Devulder J, De Colvenaer L, Rolly G, et al. Spinal cord stimulation in chronic pain therapy. *Clin J Pain* 1990;6:51–6.

Devulder J, Vermeulen H, De Colvenaer L, et al. Spinal cord stimulation in chronic pain: evaluation of results, complications, and technical considerations in sixty-nine patients. *Clin J Pain* 1991;7:21–2.

Eisenberg E, Backonja MM, Fillingim RB, et al. Quantitative sensory testing for spinal cord stimulation in patients with chronic neuropathic pain. *Pain Pract* 2006;6(3):161–5.

Frank ED, Menefee LA, Jalali S, et al. The utility of a 7-day percutaneous spinal cord stimulator trial measured by a pain diary: a long-term retrospective analysis. *Neuromodulation* 2005;8(3):162–70.

Gonzalez-Darder JM, Canela P, Gonzalez-Martinez V, et al. Spinal electrical stimulation. Current indications and results in a series of 46 patients [in Spanish]. *Rev Esp Anestesiol Reanim* 1992;39(2):86–90.

Kavar B, Rosenfeld JV, Hutchinson A. The efficacy of spinal cord stimulation for chronic pain. *J Clin Neurosci* 2000;7(5):409–13.

Kay AD, McIntyre MD, Macrae WA, et al. Spinal cord stimulation—a long-term evaluation in patients with chronic pain. *Br J Neurosurg* 2001;15(4):335–41.

Kumar A, Felderhof C, Eljamel MS. Spinal cord stimulation for the treatment of refractory unilateral limb pain syndromes. *Stereotact Funct Neurosurg* 2003;81(1–4):70–4.

Kumar K, Hunter G, Demeria D. Spinal cord stimulation in treatment of chronic benign pain: challenges in treatment planning and present status, a 22-year experience. *Neurosurgery* 2006;58(3):481–96.

Kumar K, Toth C, Nath RK, et al. Epidural spinal cord stimulation for treatment of chronic pain—some predictors of success. A 15-year experience. *Surg Neurol* 1998;50(2):110–20.

Kupers RC, Van den Oever R, Van Houdenhove B, et al. Spinal cord stimulation in Belgium: a nation-wide survey on the incidence, indications and therapeutic efficacy by the health insurer. *Pain* 1994;56(2):211–6.

Lang P. The treatment of chronic pain by epidural spinal cord stimulation—a 15-year follow-up: present status. *Axon* 1997;71–3.

May MS, Banks C, Thomson SJ. A retrospective, long-term, third-party follow-up of patients considered for spinal cord stimulation. *Neuromodulation* 2002;5(3):137–44.

Meglio M, Cioni B, Prezioso A, et al. Spinal cord stimulation (SCS) in the treatment of postherpetic pain. *Acta Neurochir Suppl (Wien)* 1989;46:65–6.

Meglio M, Cioni B, Rossi GF. Spinal cord stimulation in management of chronic pain. A 9-year experience. *J Neurosurg* 1989;70(4):519–24.

North RB, Ewend ME, Lawton MA, et al. Spinal cord stimulation for chronic, intractable pain: superiority of "multi-channel" devices. *Pain* 1991;44(2):119–30.

North RB, Kidd DH, Zahurak M, et al. Spinal cord stimulation for chronic, intractable pain: experience over two decades. *Neurosurgery* 1993;32(3):384–94.

Quigley DG, Arnold J, Eldridge PR, et al. Long-term outcome of spinal cord stimulation and hardware complications. *Stereotact Funct Neurosurg* 2003;81(1–4):50–6.

Rosenow JM, Stanton-Hicks M, Rezai AR, et al. Failure modes of spinal cord stimulation hardware. *J Neurosurg Spine* 2006;5:183–90.

Segal R, Stacey BR, Rudy TE, et al. Spinal cord stimulation revisited. *Neurol Res* 1998;20(5):391–6.

Spiegelmann R, Friedman WA. Spinal cord stimulation: a contemporary series. *Neurosurgery* 1991;28(1):65–70.

Spincemaille GH, Beersen N, Dekkers MA, et al. Neuropathic limb pain and spinal cord stimulation: results of the Dutch prospective study. *Neuromodulation* 2004;7(3):184–92.

Tseng SH. Treatment of chronic pain by spinal cord stimulation. *J Formos Med Assoc* 2000;99(3):267–71.

van Buyten J-P, van Zundert J, Vueghs P, et al. Efficacy of spinal cord stimulation: 10 years of experience in a pain centre in Belgium. *Eur J Pain* 2001;5(3):299–307.

Van de Kelft E, De La Porte C. Long-term pain relief during spinal cord stimulation. The effect of patient selection. *Qual Life Res* 1994;3(1):21–7.

Villavicencio AT, Leveque JC, Rubin L, et al. Laminectomy versus percutaneous electrode placement for spinal cord stimulation. *Neurosurgery* 2000;46(2):399–405.

Low Back/Leg Pain (Not Necessarily FBSS)

Barolat G, Oakley JC, Law JD, et al. Epidural spinal cord stimulation with a multiple electrode paddle lead is effective in treating intractable low back pain. *Neuromodulation* 2001;4(2):59–66.

Burchiel KJ, Anderson VC, Wilson BJ, et al. Prognostic factors of spinal cord stimulation for chronic back and leg pain. *Neurosurgery* 1995;36(6):1101–10.

Hassenbusch SJ, Stanton-Hicks M, Covington EC. Spinal cord stimulation versus spinal infusion for low back and leg pain. *Acta Neurochir Suppl* 1995;64:109–15.

Hieu PD, Person H, Houidi K, et al. Treatment of chronic lumbago and radicular pain by spinal cord stimulation. Long-term results [in French]. *Rev Rhum Ed Fr* 1994;61(4):271–7.

Leibrock L, Meilman P, Cuka D, et al. Spinal cord stimulation in the treatment of chronic low back and lower extremity pain syndromes. *Nebraska Med J* 1984;69:180–3.

Ohnmeiss DD, Rashbaum RF. Patient satisfaction with spinal cord stimulation for predominant complaints of chronic, intractable low back pain. *Spine J* 2001;1(5):358–63.

Raphael JH, Southall JL, Gnanadurai TV, et al. Chronic mechanical low back pain: a comparative study with intrathecal opioids drug delivery. *Neuromodulation* 2004;7(4):260–6.

Siegfried J, Lazorthes Y. Long-term follow-up of dorsal cord stimulation for chronic pain syndrome after multiple lumbar operations. *Appl Neurophysiol* 1982;45:201–4.

Slavin KV, Burchiel KJ, Anderson VC, et al. Efficacy of transverse tripolar stimulation for relief of chronic low back pain: results of a single center. *Stereotact Funct Neurosurg* 1999;73(1–4):126–30.

Low Back/Leg Pain (Not Necessarily FBSS) in Studies with Mixed Indications

Burchiel KJ, Anderson VC, Brown FD, et al. Prospective, multicenter study of spinal cord stimulation for relief of chronic back and extremity pain. *Spine* 1996;21(23):2786–94.

Meglio M, Cioni B, Visocchi M, et al. Spinal cord stimulation in low back and leg pain. *Stereotact Funct Neurosurg* 1994;62(1-4):263–6.

Mundinger F, Neumüller H. Programmed stimulation for control of chronic pain and motor diseases. *Appl Neurophysiol* 1982;45:102–11.

North RB, Fischell TA, Long DM. Chronic dorsal column stimulation via percutaneously inserted epidural electrodes: preliminary results in 31 patients. *Appl Neurophysiol* 1977/78;40(2–4):184–91.

Sundaraj SR, Johnstone C, Noore F, et al. Spinal cord stimulation: a seven-year audit. *J Clin Neurosci* 2005;12(3):264–70.

van Buyten J-P. The performance and safety of an implantable spinal cord stimulation system in patients with chronic pain: a 5-year study. *Neuromodulation* 2003;6(2);79–87.

CRPS Randomized Controlled Trials

Harke H, Gretenkort P, Ladleif HU, et al. The response of neuropathic pain and pain in complex regional pain syndrome 1 to carbamazepine and sustained-release morphine in patients pretreated with spinal cord stimulation: a double-blinded randomized study. *Anesth Analg* 2001;92(2):488–95.

Kemler MA, Barendse GA, van Kleef M, et al. Spinal cord stimulation in patients with chronic reflex sympathetic dystrophy. *N Engl J Med* 2000;343(9):618–24.

Kemler MA, De Vet HC, Barendse GA, et al. The effect of spinal cord stimulation in patients with chronic reflex sympathetic dystrophy: two years' follow-up of the randomized controlled trial. *Ann Neurol* 2004;55(1):13–8.

CRPS Long-Term Follow-Up Studies

Aló KM, Redko V, Charnov JL. Four year follow-up of dual electrode spinal cord stimulation for chronic pain. *Neuromodulation* 2002;5:79–88.

Aló KM, Yland MI, Redko V, et al. Multiple program spinal cord stimulation in the treatment of chronic pain: follow-up of multiple program SCS. *Neuromodulation* 1999;2(4):266–72.

Calvillo O, Racz G, Didie J, et al. Neuroaugmentation in the treatment of complex regional pain syndrome of the upper extremity. *Acta Orthop Belg* 1998;64(1):57–63.

Harke H, Gretenkort P, Ladleif HU, et al. Spinal cord stimulation in sympathetically maintained complex regional pain syndrome type I with severe disability: a prospective clinical trial. *Eur J Pain* 2005;9(4):363–73.

Kemler MA, Barendse GA, van Kleef M, et al. Electrical spinal cord stimulation in reflex sympathetic dystrophy: retrospective analysis of 23 patients. *J Neurosurg* 1999;90(1 Suppl):79–83.

Kim SH, Tasker RR, Oh MY. Spinal cord stimulation for nonspecific limb pain versus neuropathic pain and spontaneous versus evoked pain. *Neurosurgery* 2001;48(5):1056–64.

Kumar K, Nath RK, Toth C. Spinal cord stimulation is effective in the management of reflex sympathetic dystrophy. *Neurosurgery* 1997;40(3):503–8.

Robaina FJ, Rodriguez JL, de Vera JA. Transcutaneous electrical nerve stimulation and spinal cord stimulation for pain relief in reflex sympathetic dystrophy. *Stereotact Funct Neurosurg* 1989;52:53–62.

CRPS Short-Term Follow-Up Studies

Barolat G, Schwartzman R, Woo R. Epidural spinal cord stimulation in the management of reflex sympathetic dystrophy. *Stereotact Funct Neurosurg* 1989;53(1):29–39.

Bennett DS, Aló KM, Oakley J, et al. Spinal cord stimulation for complex regional pain syndrome I (RSD). A retrospective multicenter experience from 1995-1998 of 101 patients. *Neuromodulation* 1999;2(3):202–10.

Forouzanfar T, Kemler MA, Weber WE, et al. Spinal cord stimulation in complex regional pain syndrome: cervical and lumbar devices are comparably effective. *Br J Anaesth* 2004;92(3):348–53.

Hord ED, Cohen SP, Cosgrove GR, et al. The predictive value of sympathetic block for the success of spinal cord stimulation. *Neurosurgery* 2003;53(3):626–32.

Oakley JC, Weiner RL. Spinal cord stimulation for complex regional pain syndrome: a prospective study of 19 patients at two centers. *Neuromodulation* 1999;2(1):47–50.

Spincemaille GH, Barendse G, Rouwet EV, et al. Spinal cord stimulation and reflex sympathetic dystrophy. *Pain Clinic* 1995;8:155–60.

CRPS Case Studies

Ahmed SU. Complex regional pain syndrome type I after myocardial infarction treated with spinal cord stimulation. *Reg Anesth Pain Med* 2003;28(3):245–7.

Baldeschi GC, Babbolin G. A new and alternative leads positioning for complex regional pain syndrome treatment: paraforaminal stimulation. *Neuromodulation* 2007;10(1):12–7.

Burton AW, Fukshansky M, Brown J, et al. Refractory insomnia in a patient with spinal cord stimulator lead migration. *Neuromodulation* 2004;7(4):242–5.

Hanson JL, Goodman EJ. Labor epidural placement in a woman with a cervical spinal cord stimulator. *Int J Obstet Anesth* 2006;15(3):246–9.

Harney D, Magner JJ, O'Keeffe D. Early intervention with spinal cord stimulation in the management of a chronic regional pain syndrome. *Ir Med J* 2006;98(3):89–90.

Hayek SM. Four-extremity spinal cord stimulation using dual lower-cervical epidural octapolar percutaneous neuroelectrodes [Abstract]. *Neuromodulation* 2006;9(1):16.

Matsui M, Tomoda A, Otani Y, et al. Spinal cord stimulation for complex regional pain syndrome: report of 2 cases [in Japanese]. *No To Hattatsu* 2003;35(4):331–5.

Ochani TD, Almirante J, Siddiqui A, et al. Allergic reaction to spinal cord stimulator. *Clin J Pain* 2000;16(2):178–80.

Parisod E, Murray RF, Cousins MJ. Conversion disorder after implant of a spinal cord stimulator in a patient with a complex regional pain syndrome. *Anesth Analg* 2003;96(1):201–6.

Segal R. Spinal cord stimulation, conception, pregnancy, and labor: case study in a complex regional pain syndrome patient. *Neuromodulation* 1999;2(1):41–5.

Shah RV, Smith HK, Chung J, et al. Cervical spinal cord neoplasm in a patient with an implanted cervical spinal cord stimulator: the controversial role of magnetic resonance imaging. *Pain Phys* 2004;7:273–8.

CRPS in Studies with Mixed Indications

Abejón D, Reig E, del Pozo C, et al. Dual spinal cord stimulation for complex pain: preliminary study. *Neuromodulation* 2005;8(2):105–11.

Aló KM, Redko V, Charnov J. Four year follow-up of dual electrode spinal cord stimulation for chronic pain. *Neuromodulation* 2002;5(2):79–99.

Aló KM, Yland MJ, Charnov JH, et al. Multiple program spinal cord stimulation in the treatment of chronic pain: follow-up of multiple program SCS. *Neuromodulation* 1999;2(4):266–72.

Broggi G, Servello D, Dones I, et al. Italian multicentric study on pain treatment with epidural spinal cord stimulation. *Stereotact Funct Neurosurg* 1994;62(1–4):273–8.

Broseta J, Roldan P, Gonzalez-Darder J, et al. Chronic epidural dorsal column stimulation in the treatment of causalgic pain. *Appl Neurophysiol* 1982;5:190–4.

Devulder J, De Colvenaer L, Rolly G, et al. Spinal cord stimulation in chronic pain therapy. *Clin J Pain* 1990;6:51–6.

Eisenberg E, Backonja MM, Fillingim RB, et al. Quantitative sensory testing for spinal cord stimulation in patients with chronic neuropathic pain. *Pain Pract* 2006;6(3):161–5.

Frank ED, Menefee LA, Jalali S, et al. The utility of a 7-day percutaneous spinal cord stimulator trial measured by a pain diary: a long-term retrospective analysis. *Neuromodulation* 2005;8(3):162–70.

Kay AD, McIntyre MD, Macrae WA, et al. Spinal cord stimulation—a long-term evaluation in patients with chronic pain. *Br J Neurosurg* 2001;15(4):335–41.

Kumar K, Hunter G, Demeria D. Spinal cord stimulation in treatment of chronic benign pain: challenges in treatment planning and present status, a 22-year experience. *Neurosurgery* 2006;58(3):481–96.

Kumar K, Toth C, Nath RK. Spinal cord stimulation for chronic pain in peripheral neuropathy. *Surg Neurol* 1996;46(4):363–9.

Lang P. The treatment of chronic pain by epidural spinal cord stimulation—a 15-year follow-up: present status. *Axon* 1997;71–3.

May MS, Banks C, Thomson SJ. A retrospective, long-term, third-party follow-up of patients considered for spinal cord stimulation. *Neuromodulation* 2002;5(3):137–44.

Mundinger F, Neumüller H. Programmed stimulation for control of chronic pain and motor diseases. *Appl Neurophysiol* 1982;45:102–11.

North RB, Kidd DH, Zahurak M, et al. Spinal cord stimulation for chronic, intractable pain: experience over two decades. *Neurosurgery* 1993;32(3):384–94.

Quigley DG, Arnold J, Eldridge PR, et al. Long-term outcome of spinal cord stimulation and hardware complications. *Stereotact Funct Neurosurg* 2003;81(1–4):50–6.

Rosenow JM, Stanton-Hicks M, Rezai AR, et al. Failure modes of spinal cord stimulation hardware. *J Neurosurg Spine* 2006;5:183–90.

Sanchez-Ledesma MJ, Garcia-March G, Diaz-Cascajo P, et al. Spinal cord stimulation in deafferentation pain. *Stereotact Funct Neurosurg* 1989;53(1):40–5.

Segal R, Stacey BR, Rudy TE, et al. Spinal cord stimulation revisited. *Neurol Res* 1998;20(5):391–6.

Shimoji K, Hokari T, Kano T, et al. Management of intractable pain with percutaneous epidural spinal cord stimulation: differences in pain-relieving effects among diseases and sites of pain. *Anesth Analg* 1993;77:110–6.

Simpson BA, Bassett G, Davies K, et al. Cervical spinal cord stimulation for pain: a report on 41 patients. *Neuromodulation* 2003;6(1):20–6.

Spiegelmann R, Friedman WA. Spinal cord stimulation: a contemporary series. *Neurosurgery* 1991;28(1):65–70.

Sundaraj SR, Johnstone C, Noore F, et al Spinal cord stimulation: a seven-year audit. *J Clin Neurosci* 2005;12(3):264–70.

Villavicencio AT, Leveque JC, Rubin L, et al. Laminectomy versus percutaneous electrode placement for spinal cord stimulation. *Neurosurgery* 2000;46(2):399–405.

Peripheral Neuropathic Pain

Cata JP, Cordella JV, Burton AW, et al. Spinal cord stimulation relieves chemotherapy-induced pain: a clinical case report. *J Pain Symptom Manage* 2004;27(1):72–8.

Kumar A, Felderhof C, Eljamel MS. Spinal cord stimulation for the treatment of refractory unilateral limb pain syndromes. *Stereotact Funct Neurosurg* 2003;81(1–4):70–4.

Mearini M, Podetta S, Catenacci E, et al. Spinal cord stimulation for the treatment of upper and lower extremity neuropathic pain due to Lyme disease. *Neuromodulation* 2007;10(2):142–7.

Meglio M, Cioni B, Prezioso A, et al. Spinal cord stimulation (SCS) in the treatment of postherpetic pain. *Acta Neurochir Suppl (Wien)* 1989;46:65–6.

Murphy D, Laffy J, O'Keeffe D. Electrical spinal cord stimulation for painful peripheral neuropathy secondary to coeliac disease. *Gut* 1998;42(3):448–9.

Peripheral Neuropathic Pain in Studies with Mixed Indications

Allegri M, Arachi G, Barbieri M, et al. Prospective study of the success and efficacy of spinal cord stimulation. *Minerva Anestesiol* 2004;70(3):117–24.

Broseta J, Roldan P, Gonzalez-Darder J, et al. Chronic epidural dorsal column stimulation in the treatment of causalgic pain. *Appl Neurophysiol* 1982;45:190–4.

Broggi G, Servello D, Dones I, et al. Italian multicentric study on pain treatment with epidural spinal cord stimulation. *Stereotact Funct Neurosurg* 1994;62(1–4):273–8.

Kay AD, McIntyre MD, Macrae WA, et al. Spinal cord stimulation—a long-term evaluation in patients with chronic pain. *Br J Neurosurg* 2001;15(4):335–41.

Kumar K, Hunter G, Demeria D. Spinal cord stimulation in treatment of chronic benign pain: challenges in treatment planning and present status, a 22-year experience. *Neurosurgery* 2006; 58(3):481–96.

Kumar K, Toth C, Nath RK, et al. Epidural spinal cord stimulation for treatment of chronic pain—some predictors of success: a 15-year experience. *Surg Neurol* 1998;50(2):110–20.

Kumar K, Toth C, Nath RK. Spinal cord stimulation for chronic pain in peripheral neuropathy. *Surg Neurol* 1996;46(4):363–9.

Lazorthes Y, Siegfried J, Verdie JC, et al. Chronic spinal cord stimulation in the treatment of neurogenic pain. Cooperative and retrospective study on 20 years of follow-up [in French]. *Neurochirurgie* 1995;41(2):73–86.

May MS, Banks C, Thomson SJ. A retrospective, long-term, third-party follow-up of patients considered for spinal cord stimulation. *Neuromodulation* 2002;5(3):137–44.

Meglio M, Cioni B, Prezioso A, et al. Spinal cord stimulation in deafferentation pain. *Pacing Clin Electrophysiol* 1989;12(4 Pt 2): 709–12.

Nielson KD, Adams JE, Hosobuchi Y. Experience with dorsal column stimulation for relief of chronic intractable pain: 1968-1973. *Surg Neurol* 1975;4:148–52.

North RB, Kidd DH, Zahurak M, et al. Spinal cord stimulation for chronic, intractable pain: experience over two decades. *Neurosurgery* 1993;32(3):384–94.

Spiegelmann R, Friedman WA. Spinal cord stimulation: a contemporary series. *Neurosurgery* 1991;28(1):65–70.

Sundaraj SR, Johnstone C, Noore F, et al. Spinal cord stimulation: a seven-year audit. *J Clin Neurosci* 2005;12(3):264–70.

Van de Kelft E, De la Porte C. Long-term pain relief during spinal cord stimulation. The effect of patient selection. *Qual Life Res* 1994;3(1):21–7.

Phantom Limb/Postamputation Syndrome

Katayama Y, Yamamoto T, Kobayashi K, et al. Motor cortex stimulation for phantom limb pain: comprehensive therapy with spinal cord and thalamic stimulation. *Stereotact Funct Neurosurg* 2001; 77(1–4):159–62.

Krainick JU, Thoden U, Riechert T. Pain reduction in amputees by long-term spinal cord stimulation. Long-term follow-up study over 5 years. *J Neurosurg* 1980;52(3):346–50.

Nittner K. Localization of electrodes in cases of phantom limb pain in the lower limbs. *Appl Neurophysiol* 1982;45:205–8.

Phantom Limb/Postamputation Syndrome in Studies with Mixed Indications

Broseta J, Roldan P, Gonzalez-Darder J, et al. Chronic epidural dorsal column stimulation in the treatment of causalgic pain. *Appl Neurophysiol* 1982;45:190–4.

Broggi G, Servello D, Dones I, et al. Italian multicentric study on pain treatment with epidural spinal cord stimulation. *Stereotact Funct Neurosurg* 1994;62(1–4):273–8.

Devulder J, De Colvenaer L, Rolly G, et al. Spinal cord stimulation in chronic pain therapy. *Clin J Pain* 1990;6:51–6.

Fenollosa P, Pallares J, Cervera J, et al. Chronic pain in the spinal cord injured: statistical approach and pharmacological treatment. *Paraplegia* 1993;31(11):722–9.

Garcia-March G, Sanchez-Ledesma MJ, Diaz P, et al. Dorsal root entry zone lesion versus spinal cord stimulation in the management of pain from brachial plexus avulsion. *Acta Neurochir Suppl (Wien)* 1987;39:155–8.

Kay AD, McIntyre MD, Macrae WA, et al. Spinal cord stimulation—a long-term evaluation in patients with chronic pain. *Br J Neurosurg* 2001;15(4):335–41.

Krainick JU, Thoden U, Riechert T. Spinal cord stimulation in post-amputation pain. *Surg Neurol* 1975;4(1):167–70.

Kumar K, Nath R, Wyant GM. Treatment of chronic pain by epidural spinal cord stimulation: a 10-year experience. *J Neurosurg* 1991; 75(3):402–7.

Kumar K, Toth C, Nath RK, et al. Epidural spinal cord stimulation for treatment of chronic pain—some predictors of success: a 15-year experience. *Surg Neurol* 1998;50(2):110–20.

Lang P. The treatment of chronic pain by epidural spinal cord stimulation—a 15-year follow-up: present status. *Axon* 1997; 71–3.

Lazorthes Y, Siegfried J, Verdie JC, et al. Chronic spinal cord stimulation in the treatment of neurogenic pain. Cooperative and retrospective study on 20 years of follow-up [in French]. *Neurochirurgie* 1995;41(2):73–86.

May MS, Banks C, Thomson SJ. A retrospective, long-term, third-party follow-up of patients considered for spinal cord stimulation. *Neuromodulation* 2002;5(3):137–44.

Nielson KD, Adams JE, Hosobuchi Y. Experience with dorsal column stimulation for relief of chronic intractable pain: 1968–1973. *Surg Neurol* 1975;4:148–52.

North RB, Kidd DH, Zahurak M, et al. Spinal cord stimulation for chronic, intractable pain: experience over two decades. *Neurosurgery* 1993;32(3):384–94.

Sanchez-Ledesma MJ, Garcia-March G, Diaz-Cascajo P, et al. Spinal cord stimulation in deafferentation pain. *Stereotact Funct Neurosurg* 1989;53(1):40–5.

Sundaraj SR, Johnstone C, Noore F, et al. Spinal cord stimulation: a seven-year audit. *J Clin Neurosci* 2005;12(3):264–70.

Van de Kelft E, De la Porte C. Long-term pain relief during spinal cord stimulation. The effect of patient selection. *Qual Life Res* 1994;3(1):21–7.

Postherpetic Neuralgia

Harke H, Gretenkort P, Ladleif HU, et al. Spinal cord stimulation in postherpetic neuralgia and in acute herpes zoster pain. *Anesth Analg* 2002;94(3):694–700.

Meglio M, Cioni B, Prezioso A, et al. Spinal cord stimulation in the treatment of postherpetic pain. *Acta Neurochir Suppl (Wien)* 1989;46:65–6.

Postherpetic Neuralgia in Studies with Mixed Indications

Broggi G, Servello D, Dones I, et al. Italian multicentric study on pain treatment with epidural spinal cord stimulation. *Stereotact Funct Neurosurg* 1994;62(1–4):273–8.

Kumar K, Toth C, Nath RK. Spinal cord stimulation for chronic pain in peripheral neuropathy. *Surg Neurol* 1996;46(4):363–9.

Meglio M, Cioni B, Prezioso A, et al. Spinal cord stimulation in deafferentation pain. *Pacing Clin Electrophysiol* 1989;12(4 Pt 2):709–12.

Meglio M, Cioni B, Rossi GF. Spinal cord stimulation in management of chronic pain: a 9-year experience. *J Neurosurg* 1989;70(4): 519–24.

Sanchez-Ledesma MJ, Garcia-March G, Diaz-Cascajo P, et al. Spinal cord stimulation in deafferentation pain. *Stereotact Funct Neurosurg* 1989;53(1):40–5.

Shimoji K, Hokari T, Kano T, et al. Management of intractable pain with percutaneous epidural spinal cord stimulation: differences in pain-relieving effects among diseases and sites of pain. *Anesth Analg* 1993;77:110–6.

Spiegelmann R, Friedman WA. Spinal cord stimulation: a contemporary series. *Neurosurgery* 1991;28(1):65–70.

Tseng SH. Treatment of chronic pain by spinal cord stimulation. *J Formos Med Assoc* 2000;99(3):267–71.

Van de Kelft E, De la Porte C. Long-term pain relief during spinal cord stimulation. The effect of patient selection. *Qual Life Res* 1994;3(1):21–7.

Root Injury Pain (in Studies with Mixed Indications)

Aló KM, Yland MJ, Charnov J, et al. Computer-assisted and patient interactive programming of dual electrode spinal cord stimulation in the treatment of chronic pain. *Neuromodulation* 1998;1:1.

Aló KM, Yland MI, Redko V, et al. Multiple program spinal cord stimulation in the treatment of chronic pain: follow-up of multiple program SCS. *Neuromodulation* 1999;2(4):266–72.

Aló KM, Redko V, Charnov JL. Four-year follow-up of dual electrode spinal cord stimulation for chronic pain. *Neuromodulation* 2002;5:79–88.

Broseta J, Roldan P, Gonzalez-Darder J, et al. Chronic epidural dorsal column stimulation in the treatment of causalgic pain. *Appl Neurophysiol* 1982;45:190–4.

Kim SH, Tasker RR, Oh MY. Spinal cord stimulation for nonspecific limb pain versus neuropathic pain and spontaneous versus evoked pain. *Neurosurgery* 2001;48(5):1056–64.

Meglio M, Cioni B, Prezioso A, et al. Spinal cord stimulation in deafferentation pain. *Pacing Clin Electrophysiol* 1989;12(4 Pt 2): 709–12.

Meglio M, Cioni B, Rossi GF. Spinal cord stimulation in management of chronic pain: a 9-year experience. *J Neurosurg* 1989;70(4): 519–24.

Sanchez-Ledesma MJ, Garcia-March G, Diaz-Cascajo P, et al. Spinal cord stimulation in deafferentation pain. *Stereotact Funct Neurosurg* 1989;53(1):40–5.

Tsuda T, Tasker RR. Percutaneous epidural electrical stimulation of the spinal cord for intractable pain—with special reference to deafferentation pain [in Japanese]. *No Shinkei Geka* 1985; 13(4):409–15.

Spinal Cord Injury/Lesion

Buchhaas U, Koulousakis A, Nittner K. Experience with spinal cord stimulation in the management of chronic pain in a traumatic transverse lesion syndrome. *Neurosurg Rev* 1989;12(Suppl 1): 582–7.

Cioni B, Meglio M, Pentimalli L, et al. Spinal cord stimulation in the treatment of paraplegic pain. *J Neurosurg* 1995;82(1):35–9.

Laffey JG, Murphy D, Regan J, et al. Efficacy of spinal cord stimulation for neuropathic pain following idiopathic acute transverse myelitis: a case report. *Clin Neurol Neurosurg* 1999;101(2): 125–7.

Loubser PG. Adverse effects of epidural spinal cord stimulation on bladder function in a patient with chronic spinal cord injury pain. *J Pain Symptom Manage* 1997;13(5):251–2.

Nomura Y, Fukuuchi A, Iwade M, et al. A case of spasticity following spinal cord injury improved by epidural spinal cord stimulation [in Japanese]. *Masui* 1995;44(5):732–4.

Ohta Y, Akino M, Iwasaki Y, et al. Spinal epidural stimulation for central pain caused by spinal cord lesion [in Japanese]. *No Shinkei Geka* 1992;20(2):147–52.

Rogano L, Teixeira MJ, Lepski G. Chronic pain after spinal cord injury: clinical characteristics. *Stereotact Funct Neurosurg* 2003; 81(1–4):65–9.

Spinal Cord Injury/Lesion in Studies with Mixed Indications

Lazorthes Y, Siegfried J, Verdie JC, et al. Chronic spinal cord stimulation in the treatment of neurogenic pain. Cooperative and retrospective study on 20 years of follow-up [in French]. *Neurochirurgie* 1995;41(2):73–86.

Meglio M, Cioni B, Rossi GF. Spinal cord stimulation in management of chronic pain: a 9-year experience. *J Neurosurg* 1989;70(4):519–24.

North RB, Kidd DH, Zahurak M, et al. Spinal cord stimulation for chronic, intractable pain: experience over two decades. *Neurosurgery* 1993;32(3):384–94.

Tseng SH. Treatment of chronic pain by spinal cord stimulation. *J Formos Med Assoc* 2000;99(3):267–71.

Tsuda T, Tasker RR. Percutaneous epidural electrical stimulation of the spinal cord for intractable pain—with special reference to deafferentation pain [in Japanese]. *No Shinkei Geka* 1985;13(4): 409–15.

Waltz JM. Spinal cord stimulation: a quarter century of development and investigation. A review of its development and effectiveness in 1,336 cases. *Stereotact Funct Neurosurg* 1997;69(1–4 Pt 2):288–99.

Miscellaneous Indications

Butler JD, Miles J. Dysaesthetic neck pain with syncope. *Pain* 1998; 75(2–3):395–7.

Devulder J, De Colvenaer L, Rolly G, et al. Spinal cord stimulation in chronic pain therapy. *Clin J Pain* 1990;6:51–6.

Kirvela OA, Kotilainen E. Successful treatment of whiplash-type injury induced severe pain syndrome with epidural stimulation: a case report. *Pain* 1999;80(1–2):441–3.

Quigley DG, Arnold J, Eldridge PR, et al. Long-term outcome of spinal cord stimulation and hardware complications. *Stereotact Funct Neurosurg* 2003;81(1–4):50–6.

Simpson BA, Bassett G, Davies K, et al. Cervical spinal cord stimulation for pain: a report on 41 patients. *Neuromodulation* 2003; 6(1):20–6.

Vallejo R, Kramer J, Benyamin R. Neuromodulation of the cervical spinal cord in the treatment of chronic intractable neck and upper extremity pain: a case series and review of the literature. *Pain Physician* 2007;10(2):305–11.

Villavicencio AT, Leveque JC, Rubin L, et al. Laminectomy versus percutaneous electrode placement for spinal cord stimulation. *Neurosurgery* 2000;46(2):399–405.

Whiteside JL, Walters MD, Mekhail N. Spinal cord stimulation for intractable vulvar pain: a case report. *J Reprod Med* 2003;48(10): 821–3.

History

Deyo RA, Rainville J, Kent DL. What can the history and physical examination tell us about low back pain? *JAMA* 1002;268: 760–5.

Prager J, Jacobs M. Evaluation of patients for implantable pain modalities: medical and behavioral assessment. *Clin J Pain* 2001; 17(3):206–14.

Pain Map

Aló KM, Yland MJ, Charnov J, et al. Computer-assisted and patient interactive programming of dual electrode spinal cord stimulation in the treatment of chronic pain. *Neuromodulation* 1998;1:1.

Aló KM, Yland MI, Redko V, et al. Multiple program spinal cord stimulation in the treatment of chronic pain: follow-up of multiple program SCS. *Neuromodulation* 1999;2(4):266–72.

Aló KM, Redko V, Charnov JL. Four year follow-up of dual electrode spinal cord stimulation for chronic pain. *Neuromodulation* 2002;5:79–88.

Aló KM. Spinal cord stimulation for complex pain: initial experience with a dual electrode, programmable, internal pulse generator. *Pain Practice* 2003;3(1):31–8.

Aló KM, Holsheimer J. New trends in neuromodulation for the management of neuropathic pain. *Neurosurgery* 2002;50(4):690–704.

North RB, Fowler KR, Nigrin DA, et al. Automated pain drawing analysis by computer-controlled, patient-interactive neurological stimulation system. *Pain* 1992;50:51–7.

Parker H, Wood PL, Main CL. The use of the pain drawing as a screening measure to predict psychological distress in chronic low back pain. *Spine* 1995;20:236–43.

Ransford AO, Cairns D, Mooney V. The pain drawing as an aid to the psychologic evaluation of patients with low back pain. *Spine* 1976;1:127–34.

Physical Examination

Fishbain DA, Cole B, Cutler RB, et al. A structured evidence-based review on the meaning of nonorganic physical signs: Waddell signs. *Pain Med* 2003;4(2):141–81.

Prager J, Jacobs M. Evaluation of patients for implantable pain modalities: medical and behavioral assessment. *Clin J Pain* 2001; 17(3):206–14.

Villavicencio AT, Burneikiene S. Elements of the pre-operative workup, case examples. *Pain Med* 2006;7:S35–S46.

Waddell G, McCulloch JA, Kummel EG, et al. Nonorganic physical signs in low back pain. *Spine* 1980;5:117–25.

Imaging Studies

Holsheimer J, den Boer JA, Struijk JJ, et al. MR assessment of the normal position of the spinal cord in the spinal canal. *AJNR Am J Neuroradiol* 1994;15(5):951–9.

Prager J, Jacobs M. Evaluation of patients for implantable pain modalities: medical and behavioral assessment. *Clin J Pain* 2001; 17(3):206–14.

Miscellaneous

Eisenberg E, Backonja MM, Fillingim RB, et al. Quantitative sensory testing for spinal cord stimulation in patients with chronic neuropathic pain. *Pain Pract* 2006;6(3):161–5.

Frank ED, Menefee LA, Jalali S, et al. The utility of a 7-day percutaneous spinal cord stimulator trial measured by a pain diary: a long-term retrospective analysis. *Neuromodulation* 2005;8(3):162–70.

Psychological Evaluation

Beltrutti D, Lamberto A, Barolat G, et al. The psychological assessment of candidates for spinal cord stimulation for chronic pain management. *Pain Practice* 2004;4(3):204–21.

Brandwin MA, Kewman DG. MMPI indicators of treatment response to spinal epidural stimulation in patients with chronic pain and patients with movement disorders. *Psychol Rep* 1982;51: 1059–64.

Burchiel KJ, Anderson VC, Wilson BJ, et al. Prognostic factors of spinal cord stimulation for chronic back and leg pain. *Neurosurgery* 1995;36(6):1101–10.

Carlsson AM. Personality characteristics of patients with chronic pain in comparison with normal controls and depressed patients. *Pain* 1986;25(3):373–82.

Daniel MS, Long C, Hutcherson WL, et al. Psychological factors and outcome of electrode implantation for chronic pain. *Neurosurgery* 1985;17(5):773–6.

Doleys DM, Klapow J, Hammer M. Psychological evaluation in spinal cord stimulation therapy. *Pain Rev* 19979;4:189–207.

Dumoulin K, Devulder J, Castille F, et al. A psychoanalytic investigation to improve the success rate of spinal cord stimulation as a treatment for chronic failed back surgery syndrome. *Clin J Pain* 1996;12(1):43–9.

Kupers RC, Van den Oever R, Van Houdenhove B, et al. Spinal cord stimulation in Belgium: a nation-wide survey on the incidence, indications and therapeutic efficacy by the health insurer. *Pain* 1994;56(2):211–6.

Levita E, Rilan M, Waltz JM. Psychological effects of spinal cord stimulation: preliminary findings. *Appl Neurophysiol* 1981;44(1–3): 93–6.

Long DM, Erickson D, Campbell J, et al. Electrical stimulation of the spinal cord and peripheral nerves for pain control: a 10-year experience. *Appl Neurophysiol* 1981;44(4):207–17.

Nelson DV, Kenington M, Novy DM, et al. Psychological selection criteria for implantable spinal cord stimulators. *Pain Forum* 1996;5:93–103.

Nielson KD, Adams JE, Hosobuchi Y. Experience with dorsal column stimulation for relief of chronic intractable pain: 1968-1973. *Surg Neurol* 1975;4:148–52.

North RB, Kidd DH, Wimberly RL, et al. Prognostic value of psychological testing in patients undergoing spinal cord stimulation: a prospective study. *Neurosurgery* 1996;39(2):301–10.

Olson KA, Bedder MD, Anderson VC, et al. Psychological variables associated with outcome of spinal cord stimulation trials. *Neuromodulation* 1998;1(1):6–13.

Prager J, Jacobs M. Evaluation of patients for implantable pain modalities: medical and behavioral assessment. *Clin J Pain* 2001; 17(3):206–14.

Williams DA. Psychological screening and treatment for implantables: a continuum of care. *Pain Forum* 1996;5:115–7.

Minnesota Multiphasic Personality Inventory

Brandwin MA, Kewman DG. MMPI indicators of treatment response to spinal epidural stimulation in patients with chronic pain and patients with movement disorders. *Psychol Rep* 1982;51:1059–64.

Fordyce WE, Bigos S, Battie M, et al. MMPI scale 3 as a predictor of back injury report: what does it tell us? *Clin J Pain* 1992;8: 222–6.

Moore J, Armentrot D, Parker J, et al. Empirically derived pain-patient's MMPI subgroups: prediction of treatment outcome. *J Behav Med* 1986;9:51–63.

Symptom Checklist-90-R

Derogatis LR. *Symptom-Checklist-90-R: Scoring and procedures manual I for the revised version.* Eagan, NM: Pearson Assessments, 1977.

Derogatis Affects Balance Scale

Derogatis LR. *The Affects Balance Scale.* Baltimore: Clinical Psychometric Research, 1975.

Chronic Illness Problem Inventory

Kames LD, Naliboff BD, Heinrich RL, et al. The Chronic Illness Problem Inventory: problem-oriented psychosocial assessment of patients with chronic illness. *Int J Psychiatry Med* 1984;14(1): 65–75.

Romano JM, Turner JA, Jensen MP. The Chronic Illness Problem Inventory as a measure of dysfunction in chronic pain patients. *Pain* 1992;49(1):71–5.

Spielberger State-Trait Anxiety Scale and State-Trait Anger Scale

Spielberger C. *The State-Trait Anxiety Inventory.* New York: Academic Press, 1970.

Spielberger C. *Manual for the State-Trait Anxiety Inventory (STAI).* Palo Alto, CA: Consulting Psychologists Press, 1983.

Spielberger CD, Johnson EH, Russell EF, et al. The experience and expression of anger: construction and validation of an anger expression scale. In: Chesney MA, Rosenman RH, ed., *Anger and hostility in cardiovascular and behavioral disorders.* Washington DC: Hemisphere Publishing Corp, 1985:5–30.

Beck Depression Inventory

Beck A, Steer RA, Garbin M. Psychometric properties of the BDI: twenty-five years of evaluation. *Clin Psychol Rev* 1988;8(1): 77–100.

Beck AT, Ward CH, Mendelson M, et al. An inventory for measuring depression. *Arch Gen Psychiatry* 1961;4:561–71.

Novy DM, Nelson DV, Berry LA, et al. What does the Beck Depression Inventory measure in chronic pain? A reappraisal. *Pain* 1995;61:261–71.

Locus of Control Scale

Lau RR, Ware JF Jr. Refinements in the measurement of health-specific locus-of-control beliefs. *Med Care* 1981;19(11):1147–58.

Wallston BS, Wallston KA, Kaplan GD, et al. Development and validation of the Health Locus of Control (HLC) Scales. *J Consult Clin Psychol* 1976;44:580–5.

Absorption Scale

Tellegren A, Atkinson G. Openness to absorbing and self-altering experiences ("absorption"), a trait related to hypnotic susceptibility. *J Abnorm Psychol* 1974;83:268–77.

McGill Pain Questionnaire

Melzack R. The McGill Pain Questionnaire: major properties and scoring methods. *Pain* 1975;1:277–99.

Turk DC, Rudy TE, Salovey P. The McGill questionnaire reconsidered: confirming the factor structure and examining appropriate uses. *Pain* 1985;21:385–97.

Social Support Questionnaire

Sarason IG, Levine HM, Barsham RB, et al. Assessing social support: The Social Support Questionnaire. *J Pers Soc Psychol* 1983;44: 127–39.

Sickness Impact Profile

Bergner M, Bobbitt RA, Carter WB, et al. The Sickness Impact Profile: development and final revision of a health status measure. *Med Care* 1981;19:787–805.

Oswestry Disability Index

Fairbank JC, Davies JB, Couper J, et al. The Oswestry Low Back Pain Disability Questionnaire. *Physiotherapy* 1980;66:271–3.

Roland Morris Questionnaire

Gronbald M, Jarvinen E, Hurri H, et al. Relationship of the Pain Disability Index (PDI) and the Oswestry Disability Questionnaire (ODQ) with three dynamic physical tests in a group of patients with chronic low back and leg pain. *Clin J Pain* 1994;10: 197–203.

Fear-Avoidance Belief Questionnaire

Waddell G, Newton M, Henderson I, et al. A Fear-Avoidance Beliefs Questionnaire (FABQ) and the role of fear-avoidance in chronic low back pain and disability. *Pain* 1993;52:157–68.

Appendix A

Sample Letter of Medical Necessity for Spinal Cord Stimulation

Date

    Patient: [Patient Name]

    Policy Holder: [Patient Name]

Third Party Payer

Address   Member #   DOB:

Dear Sir/Madam:

This letter is to request a predetermination of coverage or prior authorization for the implantation of a XXXXX spinal cord stimulation system for the control of chronic pain. Spinal cord stimulation therapy is a neurostimulation pain therapy that uses epidural electrical stimulation to generate paresthesia in the area(s) of pain. It involves implanting a stimulating lead(s) near the spinal cord. The lead is connected to an implantable neurostimulator.

Spinal cord stimulation therapy does not damage the spinal cord or nerves and is considered to be a "reversible" therapy. The success of the therapy can be assessed with a trial test before permanent implantation.

Spinal cord stimulation therapy should not be confused with transcutaneous electrical nerve stimulation (TENS), which has no implantable components and acts only on the peripheral nervous system. Spinal cord stimulation therapy has been widely used since the 1970s.

Based on my review, I believe that my patient, [patient name], is an excellent candidate for this therapy.

Sample of Current Findings and Patient Status:

Mr./Ms. XXXXX has had back and radiating leg pain since October 2005, when a transport vehicle struck him/her. Imaging studies reveal right L-XX paracentral disk herniation and Lx-Lx degenerative disk disease. Mr./Ms. XXXX is currently taking oral opioids for pain control, and his/her dose has been stable for the past year. Although the medication allows him/her to work part time, he/she has great difficulty sitting, performing housework and yard work, and exercising. The majority of the pain is in the right leg. He/She has undergone lumbar epidural steroid injections with good but time-limited results.

Because [patient name] meets the patient-selection criteria and has not responded to other measures, I recommend a trial test of spinal cord neurostimulation. The decision to implant the [name of system] system will be based on the patient's positive response to the trial test, as indicated by a marked decrease in pain, improvement in function, or both.

I request confirmation that this therapy is a covered benefit, given its medical necessity, and that associated professional fees for the surgery and follow-up will be covered. I request authorization for all costs associated with the trial test and the possible subsequent permanent implant procedure, including physician professional fees and facility fee. The charge for the simulation system is included in the facility fees. The trial test has been scheduled at [name of the facility] for [date], and the permanent implant procedure has been tentatively scheduled at [name of the facility] on [date].

Thank you for your review of this information and for your coverage consideration. If you have any questions, please contact me.

Sincerely,

_____, MD

Appendix B

Frequently Asked Questions About Spinal Cord Stimulation

1. **What is a spinal cord stimulator?**

   A spinal cord stimulator is a specialized piece of medical equipment that stimulates nerves with mild electrical impulses through small electrical leads placed close to the spinal cord.

2. **Am I a candidate for spinal cord stimulation?**

   Currently, spinal cord stimulation is offered to patients with chronic and severe neuropathic pain (pain caused from damaged nerves) who have not received adequate pain relief with other treatments, such as physical therapy, psychotherapy, medications, or injections.

3. **Who should not have this procedure?**

   If you are taking a blood-thinning medication (Coumadin or in some cases aspirin) or if you have an active infection, you should not have the procedure.

4. **How does spinal cord stimulation work?**

   Spinal cord stimulation interrupts some of the painful nerve impulses to the brain. In most cases, it does not block all of the painful impulses.

5. **Will spinal cord stimulation fix whatever is causing my pain?**

   Spinal cord stimulation does not "fix" any anatomic damage that may cause pain. It can, however, decrease your pain.

6. **How will I know if spinal cord stimulation will help me?**

   It is difficult to predict whether or not spinal cord stimulation will help you. Therefore, we usually perform the procedure in two stages. In the first stage, we will place temporary leads close to the spinal cord. An external pulse generator will allow you to adjust the electrical stimulation that controls your pain.

   The trial period usually lasts from 4 to 7 days, during which you will go about your usual activities at home and work to see how well this treatment reduces your pain and affects function under normal circumstances. If stimulation relieves at least 50% of your pain, we often recommend permanently implanting the pulse generator in a second surgery.

7. **How long does the procedure take?**

   Both the trial and permanent implant can each take up to 3 hours, depending on your particular situation.

8. **What happens during the procedure?**

   The trial procedure is performed in the outpatient pain clinic. You will lie on your stomach for the entire procedure. We will monitor your heart rate with electrodes taped to your chest, your blood pressure with a cuff on your arm, and the oxygen level of your blood with a small monitor that clips to the end of one finger. We will clean the implantation site with an antiseptic solution, place sterile drapes, inject a local anesthetic to numb the skin and deeper tissues, and then perform the procedure.

   During the procedure, we will insert two thin wires or leads close to your spine through two small puncture holes. The leads will then be connected to the pulse generator. We will determine where the leads should be positioned by how much pain relief you feel at each position.

   Permanent stimulator implantation is performed in the operating room, but most patients usually go home on the same day. Some patients, however, may need to be kept overnight for observation.

9. **What are the risks and side effects?**

   Generally speaking, the surgery is safe and uneventful. However, any surgery has risks, side effects, and the possibility of complications. Please let us know your concerns beforehand so we can answer your questions.

10. **Will the procedure hurt?**

You may feel mild discomfort at first. With a small needle, we inject a local anesthetic that will numb your skin and deeper tissues, and it takes a moment for the anesthetic to take effect. Most patients also receive sedation and pain-relieving medications through an IV to help them relax, which makes the procedure even easier to tolerate.

11. **Will I be "put out" for this procedure?**

No. The leads are placed under local anesthesia as described above. You will be sedated more heavily if you receive a permanent stimulation system.

12. **Where are the leads inserted? Where is the pulse generator placed?**

For the pain involving the lower back, legs, or feet, the leads are inserted in the middle of the lower back, and the pulse generator is often placed in either the left or right upper buttock. The battery may also be placed in the abdominal area in certain patients.

For the pain involving neck, arms, or hands, the leads are inserted in the middle of the upper back. The pulse generator is often placed in the axillary region under the armpit or in either the left or right upper buttock.

13. **What should I expect after the procedure?**

You may have soreness for a day or two from the needle insertions. You should experience a tingling sensation in the areas where you normally experience pain, which is the stimulator at work. Ideally you will experience reduced pain for the duration the trial.

14. **What should I do after the procedure?**

You should arrange to have someone drive you home after either the trial or the permanent implant procedure. We advise patients to take it easy for a day or so after the procedure to heal and to allow the inflammation to subside. Activities can then be performed as tolerated with limitations on bending and stretching for 4-6 weeks following permanent implantation. If you have any questions about what activities are safe or not safe to perform, ask us; call (XXX) XXX-XXXX.

15. **How long will the battery in the pulse generator last?**

Pulse generators with rechargeable batteries are now widely available. Rechargeable batteries will last 5 to 9 years, depending on the model and manufacturer. If you do not have a unit with a rechargeable battery, the battery will need to be replaced in an outpatient surgical procedure that takes about 1 hour. Life expectancy for a nonrechargeable battery depends on how often you use it and on the intensity of stimulation required to relieve your pain. The longer it is used, and the stronger the intensity, the shorter the battery life. The useful life of the battery can thus be as short as 1 year or as long as 5 years.

Living with a Spinal Cord Stimulator

1. **Are there things I can't do?**

Yes. You will not be able to undergo MRI, therapeutic ultrasound diathermy, or microwave or short-wave diathermy once the stimulator is permanently implanted. Most SCS leads do not contain enough ferrous (iron-containing) material to be significantly affected by the static magnetic field induced in a MRI. However, the gradient magnet fields and radiofrequency fields from MRI (both pulsed during imaging) can cause device malfunction or failure by induced currents caused by rapid changes in the magnetic field or thermal and electrical burns as a result of RF-induced currents. Additionally, devices that have a magnetic (reed) switch may be activated, causing the device to reset, potentially affecting therapy.

2. **Can I go through the metal detectors at the airport?**

Yes, but the leads and pulse generator may set off the alarm. We will give you an identification card that you should present to the security guard before you go through the detectors.

3. **Can I drive?**

Yes, but you should never drive or operate heavy equipment with the stimulator turned on because it can impair your ability to control the hand or foot pedals.

4. **Where can I get additional information?**

We will give you a patient education booklet on spinal cord stimulation before you decide to have a trial of stimulation. More detailed information is available from the manufacturer of your stimulator, usually on the manufacturer's Web site.

Appendix C

Checklist of Patient Education Topics

Goals, Benefits, and Risks of SCS Therapy

Potential Therapeutic Benefits

- Pain reduction, not pain elimination (with multiple measures of pain relief considered)
- Reduced utilization of healthcare resources
- Increased activities of daily living
- Enhanced quality of life
- Decrease in symptoms of depression
- Return to employment
- Decreased medication use, with improved cognitive function

Possible Surgical Risks

- Spinal cord injury
- Infection
- Bleeding
- Cerebrospinal fluid leakage
- Paralysis

Hardware Problems

- Equipment malfunction may prevent pain relief in some patients.

Unfounded Fears Associated with SCS Therapy

- "SCS will damage the spinal cord." Clinically appropriate neurostimulation will not damage the spinal cord.

- "SCS will cause pain." SCS produces a tingling sensation, not pain.

System Operation

Ask the patient to demonstrate operation of the system. Specifically, the patient should be able to:

- Operate the programming unit after the trial implant
- Operate the control magnet and handheld programmer or transmitter after the permanent implant
- Optimize battery life
- Identify potential SCS system problems

What to Expect During the Trial Implant Procedure

The physician should cover the following topics:

- Working with the patient to select an SCS system (rechargeable vs. nonrechargeable battery)
- Preoperative restrictions and preparation
- Intraoperative procedures (including positioning), sensations, and patient expectations
- Cooperation with the healthcare team during intraoperative test stimulation by articulating response to stimulation at different lead positions
- Post-implant recovery and precautions
- Stimulation sensations after implantation (patients should know that they may become more aware of other pain once their primary pain is relieved)

**What to Expect During the
Post-Implant Period**

The physician should cover the following topics:

- Support from healthcare team members such as the physician, nurse, psychologist, workers' compensation representative, physical therapist, and other team members

- Self-care responsibilities critical to SCS treatment effectiveness, including post-implant activity restrictions
- Importance of open communication with the healthcare team regarding pain history, response to treatment, relevant psychosocial factors, and other related issues
- Importance of working closely with the clinician to achieve optimal pain relief over 6 to 8 weeks after permanent implantation.

3

Radiation Safety

In spinal cord stimulation (SCS) procedures, fluoroscopy is used to guide the insertion of needles and to facilitate directing stimulator leads. These procedures often require the use of ciné (real-time) fluoroscopy, which can potentially expose the patient and physician to significant radiation if not performed correctly. The safe use of fluoroscopy requires an understanding of the principles of safe and effective use of radiation. This information includes issues related to physics, biology, engineering, and law. This chapter provides an overview of these topics.

Background

Terminology

Measures of radiation are often expressed in both conventional units and in the more recently developed Système International d'Unités (SI; Table 3.1). Thus, exposure is a quantity of radiation expressed in the conventional units of roentgens (R), as well as the SI unit of coulombs per kilogram (C/kg). The energy absorbed from radiation, depending on the absorbing medium, is conventionally expressed as radiation absorbed dose (rad) and in SI units as grays (Gy).

However, different types of radiation with similar absorbed doses can produce dissimilar biologic effects. To predict biologic effects, as well as occupational exposure from different types of radiation, the radiation absorbed dose is converted to the radiation equivalent man (rem), or sievert (Sv) in the SI system. A quality factor (QF) is employed to account for the variable impact of specific types of radiation on biologic tissues: the radiation absorbed dose multiplied by the quality factor gives the radiation equivalent (rad × QF = rem). For example, the quality factor for x-ray radiation is 1, whereas the quality factor of alpha (He2+) radiation is about 20.

Because the quality factor is 1 for x-rays, the radiologic units of exposure, dose, and dose equivalent can be considered equal for all practical purposes, where 1 R ≅ 1 rad ≅ 1 rem, although they have different applications and meanings.

Another critical part of working with radiation is related to shielding. Shielding is usually gauged by the amount of protection that reduces exposure from a radiation source by one half. This unit is termed the half-value layer, which depends on both the energy of the radiation and the atomic number of the absorbing material. Although this exact terminology may not be clinically relevant, it is part of the lexicon that describes interactions of x-rays with shielding materials.

Radiation

Radiation is the process by which energy, in the form of waves or particles, is emitted from a source. Electromagnetic radiation has no mass and no charge. Its spectrum consists of gamma rays, x-rays, ultraviolet visible light, infrared, radar, microwaves, and radio waves (in increasing order of wave length).[1] As x-rays pass through matter, they remove electrons (ionizing radiation) from atoms, producing ionized atoms and free radicals (atoms with an unpaired electron in the outer shell), which in turn can produce harmful biologic effects. Ionizing radiation is generally classified as particulate (i.e., protons, alpha-particles) or electromagnetic (i.e., x-rays, gamma-rays).

Typical radiation levels received by an individual are estimated to average about 3.6 mSv per year or 360 mrem per year (see Table 3.1). Of this amount, approximately 85% is unavoidable background radiation and about 15% is exposure to medical radiation.[2] Although this average yearly exposure may seem small, an individual undergoing a medical procedure can potentially receive a radiation dose many orders of magnitude greater.

There are two important ways in which x-rays interact with matter. The Compton effect occurs when an incident x-ray

Table 3.1

Units of Radiation Exposure and Dose

Term	Traditional Units	SI Units	Unit Conversion
Exposure	roentgen (R)	coulomb/kg (C/kg)	$1R = 2.58 \times 10^{-4}$ C/kg
Radiation absorbed dose	rad	gray (Gy)	100 rad = 1 Gy
Radiation equivalent man	rem	sievert (Sv)	100 rem = 1 Sv

SI, Système International d'Unités.

Fishman SM, Smith H, Meleger A, et al. Radiation safety in pain management. *Reg Anest Pain Med* 2002;27(3):347–62.

interacts with a loosely bound, outer-shell electron of an atom of an absorbing material. Part of the x-ray energy is transferred to the electron as kinetic energy, causing it to eject from the atom. The x-ray is then deflected or scattered from its original path and proceeds with less energy.[1]

The photoelectric effect occurs when an x-ray interacts with a tightly bound, inner-shell electron, transferring all of its energy, some of which is used to overcome the binding energy of the electron and ejecting it. An outer-shell electron then occupies the now-vacant inner shell. This transition produces an x-ray emission called secondary radiation.

Scattered radiation from the Compton effect and secondary radiation from the photoelectric effect do not contribute any diagnostic value to the radiographic image,[1] but they do represent a radiation hazard to individuals assisting in an x-ray imaging procedure. Protecting patients and operators from scattered radiation is thus necessary, as discussed later.

In radiography, x-rays pass through the body, producing the x-ray image on a digital or film surface. In the clinical setting, x-rays are generated by an x-ray tube. The tube consists of a heated cathode close to a "target" anode. High voltage (120,000 V or 120 kVp) applied between the cathode and anode results in electrons "blasting" the anode to produce x-rays. The total flow of electrons is the tube current (mA). The quality and quantity of x-rays produced varies with the voltage (kilovolt peak [kVp]) and current (mA).

As x-rays pass through the patient and enter the image intensifier, they are converted to a visible light image that can be displayed on a television monitor or transferred to film.

Increased voltage (kVp) results in electrons with greater acceleration and higher energy. The total x-ray output is determined by the tube current (mA). Increased tube current (mA) results in an increased number of electrons striking the target. One can think of x-ray energy as being determined by both the tube current and kilovolt peak. In general, a 15% increase in voltage has roughly an equivalent effect on image brightness as doubling the tube current.

It is essential to spare the patient any unnecessary radiation exposure during fluoroscopy. Restricting the x-ray radiation exposure field through collimation restricts the x-ray beam to the required area of the body and also decreases scatter radiation and improves image quality.

Two types of collimators are present on fluoroscopes. The adjustable collimator consists of large lead shutters that are adjusted manually and that produce a rectangular field. The variable aperture collimator (or the iris collimator) restricts the fluoroscopic beam to the input field of view (Fig. 3.1). The iris collimator has smaller lead shutters that are automatically adjusted to the useful field of view (magnification and non-magnification modes) and that produce a circular field.

X-ray units are equipped with aluminum sheets that filter exiting x-ray beams. Filtration reduces the patient's radiation exposure by removing the low-energy x-rays before they have a chance to reach the patient. Low-energy x-rays are absorbed by the patient's body and do not contribute to generating an image.

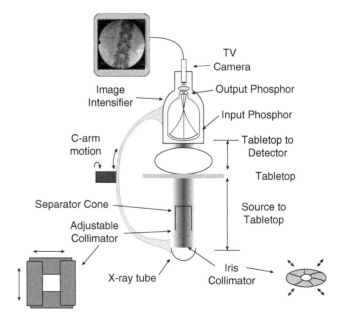

Figure 3.1 General components of the C-arm fluoroscope emphasizing differential collimation.
Note: The larger lead mobile shutters that make up the adjustable collimator are adjusted manually and produce a rectangular effect, and the smaller lead shutters of the iris collimator are automatically adjusted to the useful field of view (in magnification and nonmagnification modes), producing a circular effect.
Reprinted with permission from Fishman SM, Smith H, Meleger A, et al. Radiation safety in pain management. *Reg Anest Pain Med* 2002;27(3):347–62, with permission from Elsevier.

Image Quality

Image quality is a matter of perception that can vary between individuals. Modern fluoroscopy units typically employ an automatic brightness control (ABC) that automatically adjusts the kilovolt peak and tube current to yield optimal image contrast, brightness, and resolution.[3] Practitioners may wish to adjust voltage and current separately. Adjusting the kilovolt peak affects the image contrast by reducing the attenuation differences between different tissues (e.g., bone and soft tissue). Increased kilovolt peak decreases the contrast and increases the overall penetrability of the x-ray beam, increasing the brightness. Higher kilovolt peak values produce brighter pictures.

Lower kilovolt peak values yield higher tissue contrast. The sharpness of small structures on the fluoroscopic image is referred to as image detail. Three variables can improve image detail: (1) decreasing the distance between the patient and the image intensifier, (2) using x-ray beam collimation, and (3) decreasing kilovolt peak values.

Generally, high kilovolt peak with low tube current is preferred in fluoroscopy to produce reasonable quality images with low patient radiation exposure. Adjusted to the same image brightness, a high kilovolt peak and a low tube current expose the patient to substantially less radiation than a low kilovolt peak and a high tube current. An equally bright image can be obtained by adjusting either the kilovolt peak or the tube current. Since increasing the kilovolt peak by 15% results in the same degree of image brightening as doubling the tube current, it is safest to adjust the kilovolt peak. Increasing kilovolt peak produces much less increase in absorbed dose for the same increase in brightness.[1]

Distortion Errors

Parallax Error

Parallax error is by far the most common distortion error encountered in fluoroscopy. It is important to be sure that the x-ray beam is aligned and perpendicular to the target in all planes and centered in the middle of the image intensifier. Radiologists refer to this alignment as an orthogonal view having a set of mutually perpendicular axes, meeting at right angles. If the image is not centered and aligned, the actual target may not be where it appears to be, similar to a framing error when using a camera with a viewfinder. What is seen through the viewfinder may not be precisely what is seen by the lens.

Vignetting

Fluoroscopic images usually have less sharpness in the periphery of the image, an effect termed *vignetting*.[1] Vignetting describes the decreased spatial resolution and brightness falloff at the periphery of the fluoroscopic image. Placing the anatomic structure in question at the center of the x-ray field reduces this undesirable effect.

Pincushion Distortion

Another common effect is pincushion distortion (Fig. 3.2), which results from the detection of x-rays on a spherical surface (the input phosphor). This distortion produces somewhat of a "fish-eye" effect when the resultant electron beams emanating from a spherical surface (the input phosphor) are projected onto a flat planar surface (the output phosphor). The effect is similar to a spherical pincushion with pins that splay outward toward the edges, and it distorts the image by stretching it toward its edges.

Biologic Effects of Radiation

The biologic effects of radiation from fluoroscopy depend primarily on the dose, duration, and distance. Low doses of radiation can harm human tissues; however, normal repair mechanisms probably make most of these effects inconsequential. Nonetheless, it is conceivable that any dose of radiation can alter molecular structures and thus contribute to carcinogenesis. Dose and duration are additive and together determine the radiation exposure. Greater exposure to radiation implies greater risk (Table 3.2).[4]

No amount of radiation can be considered safe for living matter. The maximum permissible dose (MPD) is the highest

Figure 3.2 The pincushion distortion effect. *Note*: The curved input phosphor is mapped to the planar output phosphor, distorting the periphery of the image. Reprinted with permission from Fishman SM, Smith H, Meleger A, et al. Radiation safety in pain management. *Reg Anest Pain Med* 2002;27(3):347–62, with permission from Elsevier.

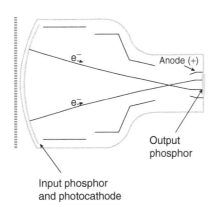
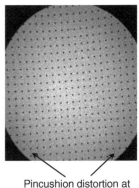

Input phosphor and photocathode

Pincushion distortion at periphery of image

Table 3.2

Annual Maximum Permissible Radiation Dose by Target Area or Organ

Target Area or Organ	Annual Maximum Permissible Dose, Traditional Unit (SI Unit)
Thyroid	50 rem (500 mSv)
Arms or legs	50 rem (500 mSv)
Lens of the eye	15 rem (150 mSv)
Gonads	50 rem (500 mSv)
Whole body	5 rem (50 mSv)
Fetus	0.5 rem (5 mSv)

SI, Système International d'Unités

Note: The International Committee on Radiation Protection recommended in 1991 that the maximum permissible dose be 2 rem (20 mSv) per year. Ideally, most radiation workers should not receive more than 10% of the MPD per year. Fishman SM, Smith H, Meleger A, et al. Radiation safety in pain management. *Reg Anest Pain Med* 2002;27(3):347–62.

dose that can be received without greatly increasing the risk of clinically important adverse effects. A radiation dose below this level probably carries only remote chances of clinically important adverse effects (Table 3.3).[5,6]

The International Committee on Radiation Protection recommended in 1991 that 2 rem (20 mSv) per year represents the MPD (see Table 3.3). The majority of the radiation exposure to the fluoroscopist is in the form of scattered radiation. The primary source of scattered radiation is the patient. Scattered exposure level is approximately 0.1% of the patient's skin entrance exposure. Assuming that proper technique and equipment are used and that the clinician is more than 1 m away from the patient, the scattered radiation exposure to the practitioner for a procedure performed under fluoroscopic guidance can be as low as 3 mR for every 1 minute of fluoroscopy time.[3]

Table 3.3

Minimum Pathologic Radiation Dose and Its Effects, by Target Organ

Target Organ	Minimum Pathologic Radiation Dose[a]		Effect
	rad	grays	
Eye lens	200	2	Cataract formation
Skin	500	5	Erythema
Skin	700	7	Permanent alopecia
Whole body	200–700	2–7	Death from infection secondary to hematopoietic failure (4–6 wks)
Whole body	700–5,000	7–50	Death from gastrointestinal failure (3–4 d)
Whole body	5,000–10,000	50–100	Death from cerebral edema (1–2 d)

[a] Minimum dose that may produce harm (e.g., cataract, permanent alopecia). Fishman SM, Smith H, Meleger A, et al. Radiation safety in pain management. *Reg Anest Pain Med* 2002;27(3):347–62.

Although this exposure is relatively small, it should not lull one into a false sense of security, particularly because radiation dose is cumulative.

The typical exposure from C-arm fluoroscopy in the average pain clinic is likely to be much less than that from fixed fluoroscopy, which is used in coronary angiography. However, the use of ciné fluoroscopy in lead placement for SCS can result in exposure rates that are much higher than those observed in typical interventional pain procedures.

Radiation exposure from fluoroscopy is not trivial (see Table 3.2). Entrance skin exposure rates generally range from 1 to 10 R per minute but can be as high as 40 R per minute with continuous ciné operating modes.[3] Under "normal" fluoroscopy conditions, the maximum legal limit for entrance skin exposure is 10 R per minute. To put this amount into perspective, typical skin entrance radiation exposures for a single posterior–anterior chest x-ray, lumbosacral spine, or abdomen films are 15 mR, 250 mR, and 220 mR, respectively. In other words, 1 minute of fluoroscopy with a typical entrance exposure of 2 R per minute corresponds to roughly 130 chest x-rays or 8 abdominal x-rays. Organ doses are less than skin doses, secondary to soft tissue attenuation.

Scattered radiation is a real concern for individuals in the fluoroscopy suite. Scatter can arrive from any conceivable direction. Larger patients and denser tissues require greater radiation output to achieve acceptable image quality and result in greater scatter.

Reducing Exposure to Radiation

The Nuclear Regulatory Commission and most other radiation safety agencies endorse the concept of "ALARA": As Low As Reasonably Achievable. This standard is based on the premise that all exposures that can be prevented should be prevented.[7] The three major ways to reduce exposure to scatter radiation are to increase one's distance from the operator and the radiation source, reduce the time of exposure, and use protective shielding.

Only necessary professionals should be in the fluoroscopy suite. Health professionals should never manually hold a patient for a study. Also, everyone in the room should be wearing appropriate shielding. Before beginning to use fluoroscopy, the operator should signal that potential x-ray exposure is beginning. It is the operator's duty to maintain awareness of the individuals in the room at all times and to stop fluoroscopy to prevent unnecessary exposure.

It is critical to understand the safety advantages of proper acquisition geometry for minimizing the dose to the patient (Fig. 3.3). Maintaining the image intensifier as close to the patient as possible reduces exposure to the detector. Maintaining the x-ray source-to-tabletop distance at as large as practical substantially reduces the entrance exposure from the image intensifier detector.

Generally, the principles of appropriate radiation safety include positioning the x-ray source at least 30 cm away from

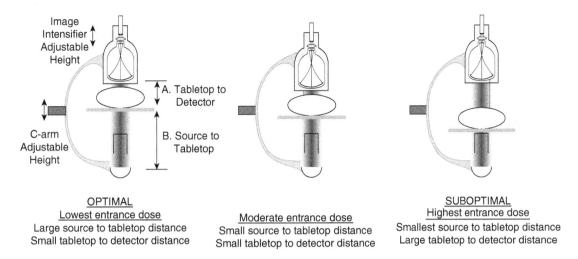

Image
Intensifier
Adjustable
Height

A. Tabletop to
Detector

C-arm
Adjustable
Height

B. Source to
Tabletop

OPTIMAL
Lowest entrance dose
Large source to tabletop distance
Small tabletop to detector distance

Moderate entrance dose
Small source to tabletop distance
Small tabletop to detector distance

SUBOPTIMAL
Highest entrance dose
Smallest source to tabletop distance
Large tabletop to detector distance

Figure 3.3 Acquisition geometry for keeping the dose as low as practical to the patient. Keeping the image intensifier as close to the patient as possible. (A) Tabletop-to-detector distance reduces exposure to the detector. A large x-ray-source-to-tabletop distance (B) substantially reduces the entrance exposure to the image intensifier detector. The least-optimal geometry is depicted on the far right, with a large tabletop-to-detector distance (A) and a small source-to-tabletop distance (B), which can increase the radiation dose received by the patient by a factor of 5 or more. Reprinted with permission from Fishman SM, Smith H, Meleger A, et al. Radiation safety in pain management. *Reg Anest Pain Med* 2002;27(3):347–62, with permission from Elsevier.

the patient; placing the image intensifier as close to the patient as is practical; positioning cone collimators down (tight) as far as is practical; and using a grid only if needed to improve image quality by reducing scatter (e.g., using geometric or electronic magnification only when necessary in large patients and relying on freeze frames as often as possible).[3]

Figure 3.4 illustrates how the electronic magnification mode allows an object to be better visualized with a smaller field of view (FOV), with its resultant increase in radiation exposure as the system compensates for lost gain. To keep the dose to the patient as low as possible, we recommend using the largest FOV appropriate for the study in conjunction with user-adjusted collimation (Fig. 3.4). Radiation exposure is inversely proportional to the square of the distance (the inverse square law)[1]—that is, as the distance from the source is doubled, the exposure rate is reduced by one fourth. Thus, maximizing the distance from the radiation source is an obvious but often overlooked means of decreasing risk. The major source of radiation is the patient, who serves as a conduit for scattered radiation. Generally, the fluoroscopic scatter exposure level from patients at 1 m is roughly 0.1% of the entrance skin exposure (e.g., if the patient entrance skin exposure rate is 3 R per minute, the operator exposure at 1 m would be about 3 mR per minute).[3] The practitioner should be aware, especially when employing a cross-table lateral view with a C-arm unit, that the amount of scatter radiation may be two to three times higher at the entrance surface of the patient (i.e., x-ray tube) than the exit surface of the patient (i.e., image intensifier).[8] Thus, standing on the image intensifier side of the patient will offer less exposure.

Minimizing exposure time includes using the least amount of fluoroscopy and ciné time possible and maximizing the use

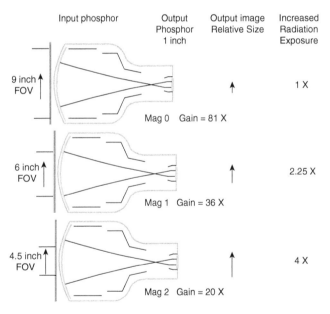

Input phosphor | Output Phosphor 1 inch | Output image Relative Size | Increased Radiation Exposure

9 inch FOV

Mag 0   Gain = 81 X

1 X

6 inch FOV

Mag 1   Gain = 36 X

2.25 X

4.5 inch FOV

Mag 2   Gain = 20 X

4 X

Figure 3.4 Minification gain. *Minification gain* in an image intensifier occurs as a result of the reduction in area of the *active* input phosphor (the field of view [FOV] to the area of the output phosphor (always a fixed diameter).
Note: This effect is equal to the square of the ratio of the input to output phosphor diameters. Electronic magnification mode allows an object to be better visualized with a smaller FOV, as shown above; however, the tradeoff is increased radiation exposure as the system compensates for lost gain. To keep the dose to the patient as low as possible, use the largest FOV appropriate for the study and user-adjusted collimation. Reprinted with permission from Fishman SM, Smith H, Meleger A, et al. Radiation safety in pain management. *Reg Anest Pain Med* 2002;27(3):347–62, with permission from Elsevier.

of the freeze-frame view, which is often described as having "a light foot on the pedal" or avoiding "lead foot." For each individual patient, the total fluoroscopy time for procedures should not exceed the "typical" time required for a standard procedure. Often, more complex or difficult procedures, such as inserting epidural leads for SCS, require use of ciné fluoroscopy, resulting in greater total fluoroscopy time. Fluoroscopic units are equipped with an automated 5-minute limit that indicates the accumulated fluoroscopic examination time and either makes an audible sound or interrupts exposure after 5 minutes of fluoroscopy.

Proper shielding is a requirement in the fluoroscopy suite. Although no law mandates the use of all the shields commonly used today (e.g., lead aprons, leaded gloves, thyroid shields, or protective eyewear), these shields are standard and essential parts of fluoroscopy, even for individuals receiving less than 5 rem (50 mSv) per year.

Preventive maintenance and quality control of the fluoroscope itself will maximize image quality and radiation safety.

Minimizing Effects on the Torso and Legs

The amount of radiation exposure to the torso can be minimized with use of a lead apron. Lead aprons absorb 90% to 95% of the scattered radiation that reaches them. There is a tradeoff between lesser weight and greater protection. For long examinations, a heavier apron can severely hamper movement, offering greater protection but potentially reducing comfort and flexibility during the procedure. "Wrap-around" lead aprons are useful for protecting the back side of the body if you will spend time turned away from the patient. If you stand near the x-ray tube, your legs should be shielded as well.

Minimizing Effects on the Thyroid

Thyroid shields are often overlooked, but they can prevent thyroid cancer. A thyroid shield should contain a lead-equivalent layer at least 0.5 mm thick.[3] As with other types of shields, greater protection also means more weight and less freedom of motion.

Minimizing Effects on the Hands

Protective hand equipment, such as x-ray–attenuating sterile surgical gloves, is recommended but provides only limited protection when within the direct x-ray field. If your hands must be protected from the beam, use densely leaded protective gloves with a thickness of at least 0.25 mm lead equivalent.[3]

Even with protective hand equipment, hands should be kept out of the beam as much as possible. Many new fluoroscopes have ABCs through which the leaded glove may be detected, resulting in increased output of radiation that negates the shielding benefit. As per Wagner and Archer: "Physicians must not be lured into a false sense of security and mistakenly rely on gloves as their principal means of protection during fluoroscopy."[3]

Use remote handling devices, such as forceps, whenever possible. Staying on the exit-beam side of the patient is also a simple and effective strategy to minimize exposure. Wearing a ring badge to measure hand exposure (white sensitive area facing palmar side) is currently the only way to assess the amount of radiation exposure specifically incident on the hands. The maximum annual hand exposure limit is 50 rem (500 mSv).[5]

Minimizing Effects on the Eyes

Protective eyeglasses with optically clear lenses that contain a minimum lead-equivalent protection of 0.35 mm may substantially attenuate scatter radiation to the lens of the eyes.[2] Leaded eyewear is recommended for individuals accruing monthly collar badge readings above 400 mrem (4 mSv). Side shields on the protective glasses, as well as a wraparound frame containing optically clear lenses with a 0.5 mm lead equivalency, are required for preventing laterally oriented scatter and are also useful for procedures that require turning your head.

Head shields are usually suspended, transparent flat plates that separate the operator from the patient and beam at approximately the operator's head and neck region. The operator works behind the shield, which can make it awkward to maneuver through certain procedures. Standing behind "lead" barriers whenever possible and keeping your head as far away from the beam as possible are good practices.

Fluoroscopy for Spinal Cord Stimulation

The use of fluoroscopy in SCS differs from the normal practice of interventional pain medicine. For conventional injection procedures, it is usually possible to take sequential freeze-frame "spot" fluoroscopy images while directing the needle incrementally. In SCS procedures, placing the Tuohy needle can also be accomplished using freeze-frame imaging; however, we have found it difficult to advance the leads without the use of some real-time fluoroscopy or at the very least frequent spot images. The challenge is to minimize exposure to both the patient and the practitioner during lead placement while maximizing the guidance afforded by live or frequent intermittent fluoroscopy.

Special training in lead handling and steering technique is required to keep the hands out of the beam when inserting the lead. In addition to the methods for reducing exposure outlined above, the beam should be directed as far as possible from the practitioner's hands during lead placement. These techniques are covered in subsequent chapters on temporary and permanent implantation. Many of the newer fluoroscopes have low-dose and/or pulse mode settings that reduce radiation output during ciné fluoroscopy. The pulse setting can often be adjusted to reduce the number of images per second. We normally set the pulse mode at 4 frames per second, which is just adequate for following the direction of the lead. A setting using fewer frames per second results in an image that is too sparse, jerky, and discontinuous. The low-dose and pulsed settings should always be used if available when live fluoroscopy is required during lead placement. The reduced resolution in low-dose mode and the flickering effect of the pulse mode usually do not interfere with the ability to visualize and direct the lead, but they do greatly reduce radiation exposure. The fluoroscopy technician should be instructed to "follow the lead" with the fluoroscopy unit as the lead is being advanced in order to continually increase the distance between the fluoroscopy unit and the practitioner's hands during lead placement. When obtaining lateral views while using a C-arm mobile fluoroscope, the operator should stand on the side of the image intensifier if possible to prevent exposure to scattered radiation as it is reflected from the patient.

Patient-Informed Consent for Radiation Exposure

An often ignored component of a fluoroscopically guided procedure is a discussion with the patient about the risks, benefits, alternatives, and other details related to radiation exposure from fluoroscopy (see Table 3.2).[3] Too often, informed consent for fluoroscopy can be overlooked or inadequate. One frequent example of inadequate informed consent involves informing the patient that fluoroscopy (or other imaging modalities) is necessary to perform an elective procedure but not that it may harm a fetus should the patient be pregnant.

The patient should be advised that radiation exposure will be kept as low as possible during the procedure. It is usually not possible to give the exact amount of radiation exposure for a specific procedure, although it is somewhere between that of a chest radiograph and angiography. The patient can also be informed that focal area exposure carries less risk than whole-body exposure.

The two major long-term potential risks of radiation exposure are the possible increased incidence of cancer and chromosomal abnormalities. The short-term effects of external beam radiation might be a skin reaction (Table 3.4). Patients should be informed that some individuals have experienced skin erythema and even second-degree burns from fluoroscopy.[9]

Questions regarding personal protection, the safety of a particular fluoroscopic suite or machine, or how to obtain additional training on radiation safety should be directed to a radiation safety officer or a qualified medical physicist.

Table 3.4
Potential Adverse Effects on Skin from Fluoroscopy

Effect	Threshold Dose (Gy)
Early transient erythema	2
Temporary epilation	3
Erythema	5
Permanent epilation	7
Desquamation and dermal atrophy	10

Fishman SM, Smith H, Meleger A, Seibert A. Radiation safety in pain management. *Reg Anest Pain Med* 2002;27(3):347–62.

Acknowledgments

This chapter is based on a previous work of one of the authors: Fishman SM, Smith H, Meleger A, et al. Radiation safety in pain management. *Reg Anest Pain Med* 2002;27(3):347–62.

REFERENCES

1. Bushong S. *Radiologic science for technologists: physics, biology and protection,* 6th ed. St. Louis, MO: Mosby Inc., 1997.
2. National Council on Radiation Protection and Measurements. Report no. 93, *Ionizing radiation exposure of the population of the United States.* Bethesda, MD: NCRP Publications, 1987.
3. Statkiewicz-Sherer MA, Viscanti PJ, Ritenour ER. *Radiation protection in medical radiography,* 3rd ed. St. Louis, MO: Mosby Inc., 1998.
4. Hall EJ. *Radiobiology for the radiologist,* 4th ed. Philadelphia: Lippincott, 1994.
5. National Council on Radiation Protection and Measurements. Report no. 116, *Limitation of exposure to ionizing radiation.* Bethesda, MD: NCRP Publications, 1993.
6. International Commission on Radiological Protection. Recommendations of the International Commission on Radiological Protection. ICRP Publication No. 60. *Ann ICRP* 1991;21(1–3).
7. National Council on Radiation Protection and Measurements (NCRP). Report no. 107, *Implementation of the principle of as low as reasonably achievable (ALARA) for medical and dental personnel.* Bethesda, MD: NCRP Publications, 1990.
8. Boone JM, Levin DC. Radiation exposure to angiographers under different fluoroscopic imaging procedures. *Radiology* 1991;180: 861–5.
9. Wagner LK, Eifel PJ, Geise RA. Potential biological effects following high x-ray dose interventional procedures. *J Vasc Interv Radiol* 1994;5:71.

4

Sterile Technique

Introduction

Despite the possibility that the following quote is both apocryphal and misattributed (to American neurosurgeon Harvey Cushing [1869–1939]), it nevertheless captures the fundamental principle of sterile technique in all invasive procedures: "Godliness is next to cleanliness."

In fact, the most important factors for preventing postoperative infections are: (1) the sound judgment and proper technique of the surgeon and surgical team and (2) the general health and disease state of the patient. In this chapter we discuss sterile technique as it applies to spinal cord stimulation (SCS) implantation and we provide background information on cleaning, asepsis, and sterilization. We describe in detail how to prepare and drape the patient for SCS implantation as well as how the surgeon should scrub, gown, and prepare for the procedure.

Remember, in the event of a wound infection following a SCS implant, the entire system most likely will need to be explanted, at great potential morbidity and cost to all. Therefore, paying close attention to sterile technique is of paramount importance.

The Importance of Sterile Technique in Infection Control

The Development of Sterile Technique

The development of sterile technique paralleled discoveries in microbiology in the 1800s, notably the introduction of germ theory by Louis Pasteur (1822–1895) and the isolation of the tubercle bacillus and the introduction of bichloride of mercury as an antiseptic by Robert Koch (1843–1910). In 1843, Oliver Wendell Holmes concluded that puerperal fever was spread by the hands of healthcare personnel. Shortly thereafter, in 1847, Ignaz Semmelweis (1818–1865) introduced the practice of routine hand washing with a chlorine solution between patients. This was the first evidence that cleansing hands with an antiseptic agent between patients was more effective than washing with soap and water in reducing the transmission of pathogens.[1]

Joseph Lister (1827–1912), the British surgeon considered to be the father of modern surgery, used a carbolic solution on dressings to prevent surgical infections and later applied the same technique to equipment and surgeon's hands. The result was a noticeable drop in mortality and evidence of a relationship between bacteria and infection.[1,2] In 1879, Lister's antiseptic techniques were formally accepted by the medical community. About the same time, in Germany, the first steam sterilizer was invented, and Gustav Neuber (1850–1932) began the practice of sterilizing everything in the operating room with mercuric chloride. He was the first to suggest that anything coming into contact with the patient should be sterile.

During this same period, surgical gowns, caps, gloves, and masks became common OR attire. William Halstead (1852–1922) of Johns Hopkins introduced rubber gloves (although primarily to protect surgeons' hands from caustic antiseptic solutions). Disposable latex gloves were not available until 1958. The gauze surgical mask, popularized by Johann Von Mikulicz (1850–1905) in 1897, became obligatory by 1926.

As knowledge of bacteriology has advanced, and the technology of infection control has improved, the principles of sterile technique have become more sophisticated and more critical. Today, a major function of perioperative personnel is to maintain an aseptic environment in the OR.

Surgical Site Infections

Sterile technique is important in preventing infection in every medical setting, but we focus here on its application in SCS implantation. Infection is the most common non–equipment-related complication of SCS implantation, so preventive measures are essential. It is devastating and demoralizing for the patient and physician to have to remove a functioning SCS system because of an infection.

Each year, 500,000 to 750,000 surgical site infections (SSIs) occur among the 30 million surgical procedures in the United States, accounting for about one-fourth of an estimated 200 million nosocomial infections.[2] The incidence of infection varies from surgeon to surgeon, hospital to hospital, one surgical procedure to another, and one patient to another. Although most of these infections are minor, about 18% lead to disabilities lasting more than 6 months, and major infections cost more than $1.5 billion each year.[2] The greatest concern with SSIs in SCS is the conduit created by the lead from the superficial pocket to the epidural space and the potential for spinal abscess formation or meningitis.

Most SSIs are associated with skin microorganisms, especially the patient's own bacteria: about 20% are caused by *Staphylococcus aureus*, 14% by coagulase-negative staphylococci, 12% by *Enterococcus* (gram-positive cocci), and 8% each for *Escherichia coli* and *Pseudomonas aeruginosa*.[2] According to data from the National Nosocomial Infections Surveillance System, the incidence and distribution of the pathogens isolated from infections have changed little over the past decade, although the number of antibiotic-resistant strains has increased.[3]

The typical person gives off 4,000 to 10,000 contaminated particles each minute. A special set of people, called "shedders," give off up to 30,000 each minute, and these particles tend to carry more virulent organisms. Not surprisingly, shedders have higher surgical infection rates.

The major areas of microbial shedding are the head, neck, axilla, hands, groin, perineum, legs, and feet.[1] In particular, hair is a major source of staphylococci; shedding is proportional to the length and cleanliness of the hair.[4] Particles from cosmetics and body powders also contain potential pathogens, as does dust.[2]

Skin bacteria are always present, despite the thoroughness of the preparation of the skin. Notably, SSIs generally result from intraoperative contamination and seldom from postoperative bacterial contamination. All surgical wounds are contaminated by bacteria, but only a minority actually become infected because the host's defenses eliminate contamination at the surgical site.[4–6]

Most microorganisms grow in warm, moist environments, but spores, some aerobic bacteria, yeasts, and fungi can remain viable in the air and on surfaces for some time.

Risk Factors for Surgical Site Infection

There are well-defined patient and surgical risk factors associated with increased SSIs:

- Patient factors[3,7–9]
  - Obesity
  - Advanced age
  - Tobacco use
  - Diabetes
  - Poor perfusion
  - Inadequately treated remote site infection
  - Systemic steroids
  - Poor nutrition
  - Prolonged preoperative stay
  - Nasal colonization
  - Perioperative transfusion
- Surgical factors[8–10]
  - Inadequate surgical field preparation
  - Shaving the operative site instead of using clippers
  - Timing of administration of antibiotic prophylaxis relative to skin incision
  - Long surgical duration (greater than 3–4 hours)
  - Inadequate hand scrub
  - OR ventilation
  - Maintenance of sterile instrument field
  - Surgical technique
  - Aseptic field (foreign material, hemostasis, sterile surgical gowning and draping technique)

Principles of Aseptic and Sterile Technique

The basis of preventing SSIs is knowing the causative agents and how they are best controlled, as well as the principles of asepsis, environmental control, and sterile technique.

Terms and Concepts

Several terms have distinct meanings in medicine but are nevertheless used interchangeably, and therefore incorrectly, in discussing sterile technique:

- **Clean** refers to the absence of visible soiling on a surface or to being free from dirt or contamination. Freshly laundered clothes, hands washed with soap and water, and mopped floors are clean; they are not aseptic or sterile unless they have undergone additional processes.
- **Aseptic**. Literally, "aseptic" means "without infection" or the absence of organisms that can cause disease. Aseptic techniques, sometimes called "clean technique," refer to methods that prevent microbial contamination of the environment. For example, the purpose of scrubbing for surgery is to render your hands and forearms as aseptic as possible. Asepsis should protect both the patient and caregiver from infection.
- **Sterile**. Technically, "sterile" is the state of being free of *all* living organisms, including spores. Some items, such as surgical tools, can be sterilized and reused, but they must be stored in sterile conditions if they are to remain sterile. However, in a "sterile operating field," the purpose of a "sterile technique" is to keep the number of microorganisms to a minimum in an otherwise clean and aseptic environment, such as a fluoroscopic suite or operating room.

- **Antibacterial activity** is measured in units of log reduction in the number of bacteria or in the percent reduction from baseline. Bacteria counts are usually very high and so are often expressed on a logarithmic scale. Thus, a $1\text{-}\log_{10}$ reduction is a reduction from 1,000 to 100; that is, by a factor of 10 or a 90% reduction. A $2\text{-}\log_{10}$ reduction indicates a reduction from 1,000 to 10, or by a factor of 100 or a 99% reduction.[1]

Cleaning and Antiseptic Agents

- **Soap** is a detergent or surfactant—a wetting agent that lowers the surface tension of a liquid, allowing easier spreading—containing esterified fatty acids and sodium or potassium hydroxide. Hand washing with soap and water can remove dirt, organic substances, and loosely adherent flora, but it has little, if any, antimicrobial activity. For example, washing your hands for 15 seconds with soap and water typically reduces the bacterial count by 0.6 to 1.1 $\log_{10}$. Repeated hand washing with soap can irritate and dry the skin, and emollients are often added to reduce these effects.[1]
- **Alcohol.** Alcohols, especially isopropanol, ethanol, and *n*-propanol alcohol, are highly effective against both gram-positive and gram-negative bacteria, including multidrug-resistant pathogens and fungi (Table 4.1). However, their effectiveness against spores, protozoan oocytes, and some viruses is poor.[1] Antiseptic solutions containing 60% to 95% alcohol are the most effective. These solutions have a rapid antiseptic effect, which declines greatly when the alcohol evaporates. Regrowth of bacteria is slow, however. Alcohol is flammable and is a fire risk if electrocautery is being used. Alcohol's antimicrobial effect comes from its ability to denature proteins.[1]
- **Iodine** is an effective antiseptic that quickly kills a broad range of microorganisms (see Table 4.1). Unlike antibiotics, iodine is not associated with the development of resistant strains of microbes. Because iodine has a strong odor and can irritate and discolor skin, iodophors—

preparations containing iodine with a solubilizing agent—are now more commonly used in antiseptic preparations.[1] A solution of povidone–iodine (Betadine) is the iodophor most commonly used as an antiseptic and scrubbing agent.[11] Iodophors are effective against gram-positive, gram-negative, and some spore-forming bacteria, as well as mycobacteria, viruses, and fungi, although they are not sporicidal in the concentrations used in medicine.[1,8] Povidone–iodine is also quickly neutralized by organic material, such as blood, irrigation solution, and pus. **WARNING**: Tincture of iodine is **NOT** the same as Betadine. Tincture of iodine is poisonous and should never be applied to a wound; it can result in the absorption of toxic levels of iodine.
- **Chlorhexidine gluconate** (CHG) is most effective against gram-positive bacteria, somewhat effective against gram-negative bacteria, minimally effective against tubercle bacilli, and ineffective against spores (see Table 4.1).[1,8] The value of chlorhexidine is its residual antiseptic activity and safety. Chlorhexidine gluconate is the active ingredient in many topical antiseptic compounds. Many hand antiseptic cleansers contain a combination of chlorhexidine gluconate and ethyl alcohol along with a moisturizing lotion to prevent chapping.[1] A single application of chlorhexidine gluconate and ethyl alcohol produces a $2.5\text{-}\log_{10}$ reduction in bacteria. Keep these solutions away from the face, eyes, ears, nose, and mouth. Combining alcohol and chlorhexidine optimizes the benefits of both substances (Fig. 4.1).[3]

Ventilation and Filtering

Between 80% and 90% of contaminants in open surgical wounds come from ambient air. Thus, surgical masks, respiratory protection, and adequate ventilation are necessary. During a long procedure, particle counts can rise to more than 1 million particles per cubic foot. Most settle on flat surfaces, especially floors. However, hot lights produce convection currents and movement stirs these particles, creating airborne contamination.[3]

Table 4.1
Characteristics of Antiseptics Used in Hand-Washing Preparations

Action	Alcohols	Chlorhexidine (Hibiclens; Avagard)	Iodine Compounds	Iodophors (Betadine)
Gram-positive bacteria	+++	+++	+++	+++
Gram-negative bacteria	+++	++	+++	+++
Mycobacteria	+++	+	+++	+
Fungi	+++	+	++	++
Viruses	+++	+++	+++	++
Speed of action	Fast	Medium	Medium	Slow
Comments	Optimal concentration: 60% to 95%; no persistent activity	Persistent activity; rare allergic reactions	Burns skin; usually too irritating for hand-washing	Less irritating than iodine; acceptance varies

Rating scale: +++, excellent; ++, good; +, fair
MMWR Recommendations and Reports, Oct. 25, 2002;51(RR16):45, Appendix: Antimicrobial Spectrum and Characteristics of Hand-Hygiene Antiseptic Agents.

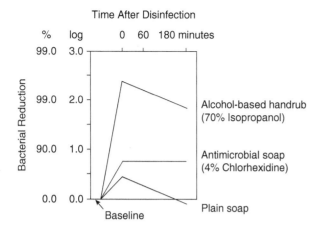

Figure 4.1 Ability of hand hygiene agents to reduce bacteria on hands. Reprinted with from *Hosp Epidemiol Infect Control*, 2e 1999. With permission from the Centers for Disease Control. Accessed at: http://www.cdc.gov/Handhygiene/download/hand_hygiene_core. ppt#338,12,Slide 12

Ventilation systems in operating rooms should provide 20 changes of highly filtered air each hour.[9] Laminar flow units can provide nearly sterile room air with a minimum of turbulence; the air flow is always in one direction.

Other Principles

In addition to cleaning and sterile techniques, several other procedures should be followed by healthcare providers to help prevent infection:

1. Bathe daily with an antibacterial soap.[3]
2. Cover all cuts and abrasions.[3]
3. Wash and rinse your hands thoroughly before entering the OR, between cases, and after removing sterile or nonsterile gloves.[9]
4. Surgical caps, gowns, masks, and sterile surgical gloves are required. Proper OR attire can reduce shedding from 10,000 to 3,000 per minute. Change into clean attire each time you enter the OR.[3]
5. Nonsterile members of the surgical team should wear long sleeves to reduce shedding from their arms.[9]
6. Reduce traffic into and out of the OR as much as possible. A lower number of people reduces the amount of bacterial shedding, and less traffic reduces air currents, which can stir up particle-borne contaminants. We block (tape a large X over) the main OR door and have people use a substerile door.[3,9]
7. Use universal precautions and treat all patients as though they had an infection.
8. Once an area is made sterile, the goal is to keep it that way. Bring only sterile items into the sterile field and move objects only from the sterile field to nonsterile areas, not vice versa. Remember that any nonsterile item in the sterile field carries the threat of infection.[9]

9. Double gloving prevents blood "strike through" on the surgeon's hands, thus helping to prevent bloodborne infections. It also reduces the risk of contaminating the surgical site by bacteria from the surgeon's hands.[3]
10. Blood and fluid breakthrough on the surgical gown, especially on the surgeon's forearms, increases the passage of microbes through the gown. Gowns that have become soaked should be replaced.[3]
11. Wet drapes on the patient may allow bacteria to pass into the operative area from other, unprepared areas. Drapes that have become soaked should be replaced.[3]
12. Wide areas of skin preparation around the proposed surgical site will reduce the risk of microbial breakthrough into the wound area if towels and drapes become wet.[3]
13. Placing plastic adherent border drapes clearly defines the area to be prepared and provides an additional barrier to the influx of bacteria from outside the field.[3]
14. Keep all sterile equipment, including the leads and pulse generator, packaged or covered until they are needed.[3,9]
15. Physically separate clean from soiled items.
16. Promptly disinfect contaminated equipment, reusable supplies, and surfaces.

Preoperative Preparation: Home Preparation

Preparing the patient for an SCS trial begins well before the surgery and involves the patient's own care. Here, we describe the preoperative preparation we use before performing an SCS trial or permanent implant.

1. Treat and control all bacterial infections in the patient before the procedure.[3,9]
2. Have the patient take a shower from head to toe with chlorhexidine liquid soap on the night before and the morning of the procedure (within 12 hours of the procedure).[1,3,11] Instruct the patient as follows:
   a. "Wet your body and hair, shampoo your hair with your regular shampoo, and wash thoroughly with your regular soap. Rinse thoroughly, then turn the water off. Cover your body from the neck down with chlorhexidine liquid. Be sure to avoid getting the soap in your face, eyes, ears, nose, and mouth. Wash your body gently but thoroughly for at least 5 minutes, then rinse. Do not use your regular soap after washing with chlorhexidine; it may bring unwanted bacteria back to your body. Dry yourself with a clean towel and do not apply powders, deodorant, or lotions. Dress in clean clothes."
   b. Note: In patients who are carriers or suspected carriers of methicillin-resistant *Staphylococcus aureus*

(MRSA), the following presurgical treatment should be considered:

- Use chlorhexidine (Hibiclens) or hexachlorophene (pHisoHex) antiseptic soap. Wash the whole body (from scalp to toes) once daily. A big lather is not necessary. A skin moisturizer may be applied for dry skin after bathing.
- Remove all artificial nails and all fingernail polish.
- Scrub fingernails for 1 minute with nail brush twice daily.
- This should be repeated daily starting 7 days before surgery.[12–14]

3. If possible, avoid shaving the surgical area with a razor, especially on the day of the surgery; small cuts in the skin can harbor microorganisms. If using a razor is required, remove hair from the surgical area no less than 7 days before the trial or permanent implant. Electric clippers are preferable because they do not actually scrape or cut the skin. Depilatory agents may be used if necessary but their use occasionally results in a hypersensitivity reaction, which can itself lead to an SSI.[3,5,7,9,11]

Prophylactic Antibiotics

Optimization of antimicrobial prophylaxis has been one of the most important advances in reducing SSIs. The fundamental concept in preventive antibiotic use is that there is a "decisive period" during which antibiotics will be effective. This decisive period lasts only a few hours, and operations should begin and end within this decisive period.

Although prophylactic antibiotics can help prevent infection in surgical patients, their effectiveness depends on:

1. Choosing the appropriate antibiotic: The antibiotic should be effective against pathogens most commonly associated with infections specific to the procedure as well as those endogenous to the region of the body involved. The Infectious Disease Society of America, Surgical Care Improvement Project (SCIP)[15] for non–intra-abdominal surgeries such as SCS procedures recommends giving a cephalosporin such as cefazolin 1 g or cefuroxime 1.5 g intravenously. If the patient is allergic to beta-lactams, substitute clindamycin 600 mg. If the patient is colonized with MRSA, use vancomycin 1 g.
2. Proper timing of antibiotic administration before surgery: Time the administration so that the concentration of the antibiotic is highest at the time of the incision. This period ranges from 30 to 120 minutes before surgery. Therefore, skin incision should not occur until at least 30 minutes after antibiotics have been administered. Antibiotics administered after surgery will not prevent SSIs.
3. Limiting the duration of antibiotic administration after surgery: Therapeutic levels should be maintained throughout the surgery. If the surgery is longer than the half-life of the drug, the drug should be readministered.

Administration should be stopped within 24 hours after surgery. Administration for longer than 24 hours postsurgery provides no additional benefit, and unnecessary administration promotes the development of antibiotic-resistant microorganisms.[5]

Operative Preparation: Scrubbing and Draping

Have the patient lie prone on the fluoroscopic table so that there is free access to the appropriate areas of the spine with the fluoroscope. Position the patient for either a cervical or lumbar implantation by placing pillows under the chest or abdomen, respectively, to optimize access to the epidural space. Place a blanket over the patient for warmth until the surgical preparation begins.

At least 30 minutes before the procedure, start an IV antibiotic drip containing one of the antibiotics listed above.

When the patient is positioned and the IV has been started, the patient may be scrubbed for surgery as follows:

1. Identify the region of the patient's back to be prepped for surgery. For placing cervical leads, the area to be prepped will extend from the hairline to the small of the back and to both sides of the table; for thoracic and lumbar leads, it will extend from the mid-scapula to the buttocks and to both sides of the table.
2. Place plastic adhesive border drapes around the area to be prepped and along both sides of the spine. Placing plastic border drapes clearly identifies the area to be prepped and provides an additional barrier from bacteria outside of the field.
3. Scrub the patient's back with povidone–iodine for at least 5 minutes. The surgeon or surgical assistant should begin scrubbing the center of the region to be prepped and move outward to the sides of the rib cage and onto the plastic border drapes. This will provide as large a sterile field as possible. The entire area should be scrubbed with several sponges for at least 5 minutes. When done, a sterile towel should be placed over the region and any extra povidone–iodine removed by blotting. We recommend that surgeons either be present for the preparation or perform it themselves to ensure that the area is properly scrubbed.
4. Apply chlorhexidine to the region. Apply a one-time application of chlorhexidine or DuraPrep by starting in the middle of the field and working to the edges. If using chlorhexidine, let the excess remain wet on the patient's back and absorb into the skin. If using DuraPrep, allow it to dry. (Note: We use and recommend a sequential preparation with povidone–iodine followed by another agent that either absorbs into or adheres to the skin to provide durable antimicrobial protection. The second compound is necessary because blood and other fluids neutralize the broad antimicrobial effect of povidone–iodine. Chlorhexidine can be used as the second preparation.

Although it has a somewhat narrower antimicrobial spectrum than povidone–iodine, it is absorbed into the skin and provides longer protection. Many implanters use DuraPrep as another alternative. It is a povidone–iodine solution that adheres to the skin to provide lasting antimicrobial protection. Dura Prep is ideally used in conjunction with a plastic adhesive film (see below). The operating surgeon should now perform a hand scrub and put on a gown and gloves before proceeding to the next steps. See below for instructions on gowning and gloving.

5. Apply four cloth-border drapes around the prepared region of the patient's back. Fold the top of the first drape over 2 or 3 inches and place the folded edge along the inside edge over the plastic adhesive border drapes of the field to cover the nonsterile side of the table. Place the second drape along the far side, and lay the third and fourth drapes at the bottom and top of the field. The weight of the drapes should keep them in place. Be careful not to touch the side of the fluoroscopic table with your gown while draping, as it is not sterile.

6. If using chlorhexidine, blot the excess from the patient's back with a sterile towel. The patient's back must be dry for the next step.

7. Cover the surgical field with a povidone–iodine–impregnated plastic adhesive incise antimicrobial surgical film (Ioban, 3M Healthcare). Incise antimicrobial surgical film is polyester film coated with medical-grade acrylate adhesive that contains molecular iodine to protect the skin from contaminating the leads, extensions, and pulse generator during implantation. (Use a non-impregnated adhesive drape if the patient is allergic to iodine.) It comes folded in a long rectangular package. Remove the wrapping and hold the edge of the sheet over the drape at the top of the field. With your other hand, pull the lower, white edge of the sheet down the patient's back, smoothing the sheet back as you pull. (The sheet unfolds from the top, making it easier to apply. Unfolding the entire sheet and attempting to lay it on the patient's back at one time is unnecessarily difficult and may result in large air bubble trapped under the sheet. This type of application is not recommended. Apply the sheet until it covers the entire field from above the edge of the top border drape to below the edge of the bottom drape.

8. Apply a U-shaped cover drape to the patient's lower back and sides. The drape comes folded in the middle. Remove the backing from the adhesive at the inside bottom of the U and fix the fold along the patient's waist so that the lower half of the drape covers the legs and feet and the upper half is folded back. Next, remove the backing from the adhesive along the arms of the U and extend the film up along the patient's sides, covering the earlier drapes.

9. Apply a final bar drape to the head and shoulders. This drape should extend from the top of the surgical field to well above the patient's head. An assistant will gather the extra material and arrange it above and around the patient's head.

10. Apply a side drape to allow lateral fluoroscopic views during the procedure. Extend the drape along the side of the patient, letting it fall over the side of the table. Attach the side drape to the other drapes with Allis clips, making sure to keep them clear of the x-ray field. Towel clips should not be used as they can puncture the drape, whereas the Allis clips will not.

11. C-arm cover: The image intensifier must be covered with a sterile clear plastic drape so that it can be maneuvered without contaminating gloves.

The patient is now scrubbed and draped for the procedure.

Physician Preparation: Hand Scrubbing, Gowning, and Gloving

We suggest that physicians performing SCS implantation prepare themselves as follows. The clinician is ready to scrub for surgery after donning clean scrubs, surgical cap and mask, eye protection, shoe covers, and a lead apron. The scrub described below should be done once in the morning and again in the afternoon, but you should reapply a chlorhexidine/alcohol hand preparation between patients if you are performing multiple procedures.

1. Remove rings and watches and wash hands and forearms with soap and hot water. The first wash should be done with running water and a water-based cleanser (soap) to mechanically remove the dirt and spores that are not removed by alcohol products. Complete the entire scrubbing procedure over a sink so that water will not drip from your hands and elbows onto the floor during the scrub.[3]

2. Begin by cleaning under each fingernail with the nail cleaner. (The plastic cleaner comes in the package.) Remove all visible debris from under your nails. Nails should be maintained short and clipped. Shorter nails are less likely to trap particles and to puncture surgical gloves. Artificial nails should not be worn.[1,3]

3. Scrub both arms up to the elbows with povidone–iodine for approximately 5 minutes. Unwrap the sponge and apply the scrub to your hands and forearms while working up a good lather. Scour your fingertips with the bristles. The bristles can irritate the skin, so reserve them for scrubbing under your nails and between your fingers, where lines and creases can harbor microorganisms. Sponge and scrub your fingertips, hands, and forearms for about 5 minutes to allow for the solution's maximum effect. Scrubbing with povidone–iodine provides both a mechanical and a chemical cleansing action, both of which are more effective when applied for the full 5 minutes.[3,8]

4. Apply chlorhexidine/alcohol solution to your hands and forearms. Chlorhexidine/alcohol solution is dispensed from a foot-operated pump. Apply the first two

handfuls to your forearms and the third handful specifically to your hands. As with the povidone–iodine scrub, spread the chlorhexidine/alcohol solution on your forearms first so it can begin its action, and then focus on your nails, cuticles, and interdigital spaces before returning to the rest of your hands and forearms. Allow the alcohol to evaporate before gowning.

5. Put on a surgical gown. If you are performing surgery in the OR, a surgical technician (scrub tech) will typically hold your gown such that you can insert your arms into the sleeves. If you are gowning yourself, the gown should come folded in a sterile package. Open the package and grip the gown by the back. Grasp the arm slits on the side of the folded gown and gently shake it open; the arm openings will appear as the front of the gown falls open in front of you. Insert your arms in the sleeves but do not yet extend your hands through the cuffs. Have an assistant close the gown behind you and secure the ties. The front of your body is now sterile, but your back is not considered sterile.

6. Put on surgical gloves. Closed gloving: If you are working in an OR the scrub tech will hold your gloves for easy insertion of your hands. Without an assistant, you will need to open the package through the sleeve of the gown. If you intend to double glove, putting darker gloves on first will make any punctures in the outer, lighter gloves more visible. With one hand, hold the glove through the sleeve, and with the other, again through the sleeve, turn the first few inches of the cuff of the glove inside out. Putting the cuff of the glove over one hand, push the hand through the cuff of the gown and into the glove; then, with your other hand, pull the folded cuff of the glove back down over your hand. Repeat the process on the other hand. Adjust both gloves until they are comfortable on your hands. The second glove is easy to apply because your hands are already sterile. Note: The inner glove should be a half-size larger than the outer glove (yes, that's right) so that they are not too tight. Wearing two gloves of the same size can cut off circulation and compress the median nerve, leading to cramping.

7. Belt the gown. On the front of the gown is a white tab that is attached to the belt of the gown. Have an assistant hold the tab while you turn around to pull the belt around you, then tighten and tie it closed.

You should now be scrubbed and gowned and ready to perform the procedure.

REFERENCES

1. Centers for Disease Control and Prevention. Guide for Hand Hygiene in Health-Care Settings. Recommendations of the Healthcare Infection Control Practices Advisory Committee and the HIPAC/SHEA/APIC/IDSA Hand Hygiene Task Force. *MMWR* 2002;51:1–45.

2. Seal LA, Paul-Cheadle D. A systems approach to preoperative surgical patient skin preparation. *Am J Infect Control* 2004:32(2): 57–62.

3. Mangram AJ, Horan TC, Pearson ML, et al. Guideline for prevention of surgical site infection, 1999. *Infect Control Hosp Epidemiol* 1999;20(4):248–78.

4. Cheadle WG. Risk factors for surgical site infection. *Surg Infect* 2006;7(1):S7–S11.

5. Nichols RL. Preventing surgical site infections: a surgeon's perspective. *Emerg Infect Dis* 2001;7(2):220–4.

6. Tavolacci MP, Pitrou I, Merle V, et al. Surgical hand rubbing compared with surgical hand scrubbing: comparison of efficacy and costs. *J Hosp Infect* 2006;63:55–9.

7. UCSF Medical Center. *UCSF medical center infection control manual: guidelines for wound care and prevention of surgical site infections.* 1992:1–8.

8. Leaper DJ. Risk factors for surgical infection. *J Hosp Infect* 1995;30:127–39.

9. Garner JS. CDC guidelines for prevention of surgical wound infections, 1985. *Infect Control* 1986;7(3):193–200.

10. Barnard BM. Fighting surgical site infections. *Infect Control Today* 2002:1–5.

11. Bjerke N, Hobson DW, Seal LA. Preoperative skin preparation: a systems approach. *Infect Control Today* 2001:1–5.

12. Haley CE, Marling-Cason M, Smith JW, et al. Bactericidal activity of antiseptics against methicillin-resistant *Staphylococcus aureus*. *J Clin Microbiol* 1985;21(6):991–2.

13. Nguyen DM, Mascola L, Brancoft E. Recurring methicillin-resistant *Staphylococcus aureus* infections in a football team. *Emerg Med News* 2005;27(3):54–9.

14. Siegel JD, Rhinehart E, Jackson M, et al., Healthcare Infection Control Practices Advisory Committee. Management of multidrug resistant organisms in healthcare settings. *Am J Infect Control* 2007;35(10):S165–93.

15. Solomkin JS, Mazuski JE, Baron EJ, et al. Guidelines for the selection of anti-infective agents for complicated intra-abdominal infections. *Clin Infect Dis* 2003;37(15):997–1005.

5

Electricity and Spinal Cord Stimulation

Introduction

It is necessary for implanters to understand the basic theory behind spinal cord stimulation (SCS) equipment, including the effects of current, voltage, and impedance on stimulated structures in the spinal column. Although the technical aspects of SCS can get complicated, implanters need not become electrical engineers.

SCS is most commonly performed using platinum alloy contacts placed in the epidural space. The contacts are attached to a catheter-style lead that is connected to a pulse generator, which provides power and programming capabilities. The generator creates a voltage potential on the contacts in the spinal column and the current generated by the voltage potential stimulates neurons in the dorsal structures of the spinal cord (dorsal column [DC] and dorsal root [DR] fibers) that can inhibit pain transmission. The patient perceives the stimulation as a cutaneous paresthesia or tingling sensation. For SCS to be successful, the paresthesia must overlap the painful area.

SCS Leads

Two lead types are currently in use—percutaneous and surgical (paddle) leads.

Percutaneous Leads

Percutaneous leads are flexible cylindrical polyurethane catheters with multiple, evenly spaced cylindrical electrode contacts arranged at the distal end. The main differences between varying types of percutaneous leads can be categorized according to the contact length, diameter/width, number of contacts, and distance between contacts. Percutaneous leads currently have 4 or 8 electrodes, but leads with 16 contacts may soon become available. The electrodes themselves are composed of platinum alloy (often platinum–iridium) and range from 3 to

6 mm in length, with edge-to-edge spacing of 1 to 12 mm depending on the manufacturer and model. Multiple contacts along the lead allow for stimulation field shaping as well as post-implant reprogramming if lead migration occurs. The cylindrical design of percutaneous electrodes allows current to flow circumferentially, creating the possibility of 360-degree stimulation. Circumferential stimulation has been implicated in painful sensations due to the likely stimulation of posterior structures in the epidural space, such as the ligamentum flavum. This argument, among others, has been used in support of the preferred use of surgical leads.[1–3]

Surgical (Paddle) Leads

Surgical (paddle) leads are flat and wide at the distal end, with up to 16 electrodes placed on one side of a flexible rectangular silicone backing. The design allows for unidirectional current flow toward the cord, and there is clinical evidence that paddle leads may eliminate discomfort due to the dorsal structure stimulation sometimes seen with cylindrical leads.[1] Owing to their shape, paddle leads cannot be inserted via a needle and must be surgically implanted via a laminotomy/laminectomy by a neurosurgeon and are therefore beyond the scope of this book.

Ohm's Law (V = IR)

Ohm's law describes the relation between voltage (V), current (I), and impedance/resistance (R). In an electrical circuit, *voltage* is the electrical pressure that pushes electrons. *Current* is the flow of electrons. *Impedance/resistance* is the characteristic of a material that resists the flow of current. In the body, impedance is determined by the electrical characteristics and composition of the tissue surrounding the contacts. Although impedance and resistance are not truly the same thing, they are analogous, and for the sake of simplicity, we can use these terms synonymously. Plainly stated, the higher the resistance, the higher the voltage required to maintain a given current flow. For an implanted pulse generator (IPG), the battery life of a nonrechargeable/primary cell-based device and the recharging interval of a device with a rechargeable battery will ultimately be determined by the power demands on the system. Since power is a function of both voltage and current, power consumption is clearly influenced by impedance, so understanding and optimizing the variables that contribute to impedance offers an opportunity to enhance power performance.

Perception Threshold

The perception threshold is a measure of the minimum stimulation pulse amplitude necessary to generate a perceptible sensation. The perception threshold is a parameter than can be influenced by either impedance and/or dispersion of current. If the impedance is increased, as in the case of increased scar tissue, the amount of energy required to reach the perception threshold is increased. In a constant-voltage stimulation system, this may require that the stimulation voltage amplitude is increased to maintain the same current. In a constant-current stimulation system, however, the voltage will automatically be increased by the system to compensate for the increased resistance from the scar tissue, and thus should theoretically not require an increase in stimulation current amplitude. If the distance from the target tissue is increased, such as by a thick cerebrospinal fluid (CSF) layer, then more energy will be required to activate the DC and/or DR fibers and the perception threshold will also be increased.

Fibrosis

The body reacts to chronically implanted foreign objects by attempting to isolate them with fibrotic scar tissue encapsulation. A fibrotic sheath inevitably forms around an implanted electrode, and electrical resistance is increased by such scar tissue formation. Evidence suggests that impedance increases by 26% on average by 3 months after implant.[4] To complicate the matter, scar tissue develops unevenly around each electrode and also changes over time (Fig. 5.1).[4] Given the variable pattern of scar formation around each lead, adjusting and redirecting current as scar tissue forms may be necessary to be able to recapture stimulation of the painful area. Several strategies, including current steering and pulse interleaving, are currently used to recapture stimulation if the paresthesia becomes discordant.

Epidural Space

The epidural space appears to be more segmented and less uniform than once believed. The ligamentum flavum is not uniform along the length of the spine or within the intervertebral space. The distance between the ligamentum flavum and the dura varies with location in the spinal column. In the upper thoracic spine the distance is approximately 3 to 4 mm, and it gradually increases more caudally in the thoracic spine.

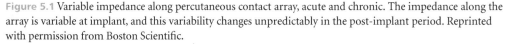

Figure 5.1 Variable impedance along percutaneous contact array, acute and chronic. The impedance along the array is variable at implant, and this variability changes unpredictably in the post-implant period. Reprinted with permission from Boston Scientific.

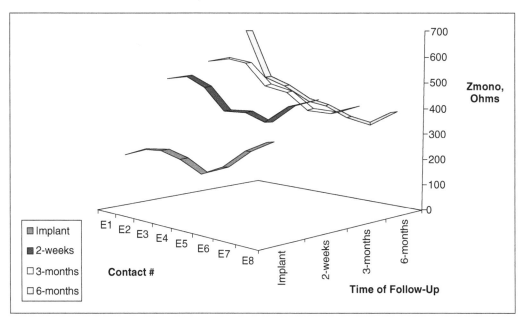

The greatest anterior–posterior (AP) distance occurs at L2 where, in adults, it measures 5 to 6 mm. From C3 to C7, the distance between the dura and ligament is quite narrow. At C7 the distance is reduced to 1.5 to 2 mm because of the enlargement of the cord at that level. Not surprisingly, it has been shown that the impedance is typically higher when a lead is placed in the lower thoracic spine as opposed to the cervical spine.[5] Given the large epidural space present in the lower thoracic space, there is no guarantee that the lead will be in contact with the dura, and a relatively dorsal position of the contacts may result in a higher impedance. Because higher impedances have been demonstrated in the lower thoracic epidural space, systems implanted in the cervical epidural space may enjoy a longer battery life than systems implanted in the thoracic region. In present clinical practice, lead placement is usually performed by optimizing only the cephalocaudal and mediolateral position of the lead. Whether new strategies will be developed to optimize dorsoventral positioning of the lead has yet to be seen. In fact, this is an argument in favor of paddle lead placement, particularly in the lower thoracic spine, since paddles can be placed directly on the dura under visual guidance. In the long run, the growth of a fibrotic layer around the lead may ultimately equalize the gross impedances seen in the cervical and thoracic regions (though not necessarily the impedance variability along the lead). In any chronic patient, this leaves the electrode-to-spinal cord distance as the dominant predictor of thresholds and thus power requirements.

CSF Layer

The perception threshold has been shown to be affected by the thickness of the dorsal CSF layer between the stimulating contacts and the cord at the level being stimulated.[6–11] CSF is an effective conductor that tends to disperse current. Such dispersion can cause current to wrap around the cord, resulting in uncomfortable lateral root stimulation, particularly at the low-thoracic level. Because of variations in spinal cord anatomy among individuals and variations in CSF thickness at different levels of the cord in the same individual, the perception threshold can vary greatly. On average, the cord diameter is inversely proportional to the CSF layer thickness. Thus, the cord diameter is usually smallest at the T3 to T6 level and the CSF layer is the greatest.[12]

Perception thresholds may be high when placing leads in the upper thoracic region over a thicker CSF layer. In contrast, when leads are placed in the midline in the upper cervical spine the threshold for stimulation is very low because of the thin CSF layer.

Time Since Implant

Elapsed time since implantation has also been shown to affect impedance. This appears to be related to the formation of fibrotic tissue. It has been shown that impedance is relatively low in the first 4 to 5 days after implantation. It may be that early edema formation resulting from minor epidural trauma around the lead lowers impedance in the early acute period. In the following weeks, the edema fluid resolves and fibrosis develops, thereby increasing impedance.[4]

Other Factors

Male gender is associated with 21% higher impedance in the lower thoracic spine than female gender. There are no anatomic data from which to interpret this finding, although the reduced epidural fat layer in females compared with males may offer a plausible explanation. Age, previous spine surgery, number of leads, and lead model have not been shown to affect impedance.[5]

Anodes and Cathodes

Modern SCS leads have multiple contacts (also referred to as electrodes) that can be programmed individually as anodes (positive polarity), cathodes (negative polarity), or off (inactive). Ideally, a contact must be made of a metal that is always nontoxic, nonimmunogenic, and noncorrosive. It must maintain its shape and withstand surgical implantation. It must also be able to effectively conduct current so that the surrounding nervous tissue is effectively depolarized. Platinum alloys meet these requirements.

In electrical stimulation, positive current is defined as flowing from the anode to the cathode. The cathode is the working electrode that causes nerves to depolarize and generate action potentials. In most cases, stimulation paresthesias result from the activation of fibers closest to the cathode level.[13] The anode is the counter-electrode that hyperpolarizes surrounding nerves, thus rendering them more resistant to depolarization (Fig. 5.2).

It is useful to understand the different nature of current conduction in the body as opposed to that in an electrical circuit. Within the IPG, electrical current is carried by free electrons in metal conductors and semiconductors. However, the current in the physiologic medium between the anode and cathode is carried primarily by sodium, potassium, and chloride ions and polarized molecules found in the extracellular fluid. An interface is formed at the surface of the electrode and within microns of the tissue adjacent to it. It is at this interface that complex chemical reactions occur (depending upon anodic or cathodic polarity) that essentially transduce the electron-based current in the IPG and lead to an ion-based current in the tissue. This interface plays a crucial role in preventing net charge transfer (leading to degradation of the electrode) by acting as an effective capacitance. As discussed below, however, this interface capacitance can also contribute to a dynamic impedance seen at the electrode during the stimulation pulse, which may influence the stimulation field in voltage-controlled stimulators.

Lateral View

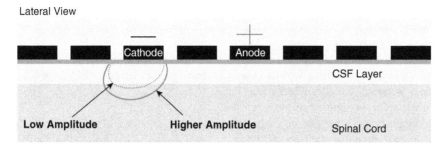

Figure 5.2 Simplified stimulation loci generated by a bipole in the dorsal columns. The main region of stimulation (aka volume of activation [VOA]) occurs beneath the cathode. At low amplitudes, only superficial fibers will be activated; as stimulation pulse amplitude is increased, the VOA will penetrate deeper into the cord, activating more fibers. At typical electrode-to-spinal cord distances and bipole lead spacings, the anode hyperpolarizes nearby tissue. The net effect of this hyperpolarization is to "push" the VOA away from the anode, thus shaping the stimulation VOA. Reprinted with permission from Boston Scientific.

Dorsal Column Anatomy

Dermatomes are cutaneous areas of the body innervated by a specific nerve root (Fig. 5.3).

A spinal nerve root is made up of a dorsal (sensory) and a ventral (motor) root. For example, the dermatome for the L4 sensory root covers primarily the medial calf. Damage to that nerve root often results in pain and/or numbness in that distribution. The dorsal and ventral roots combine to form mixed spinal nerves as they exit the spine.

The DC is composed of nerves of different diameters that perform sensory, motor, and proprioceptive functions. These nerves run longitudinally in the DC and, depending on lead location, are within range of the electrodes placed in

Figure 5.3 Nerve roots supplying cutaneous dermatomes. Reprinted with permission from Flynn JA. *Oxford American Handbook of Clinical Medicine.* Oxford University Press, New York © 2007.

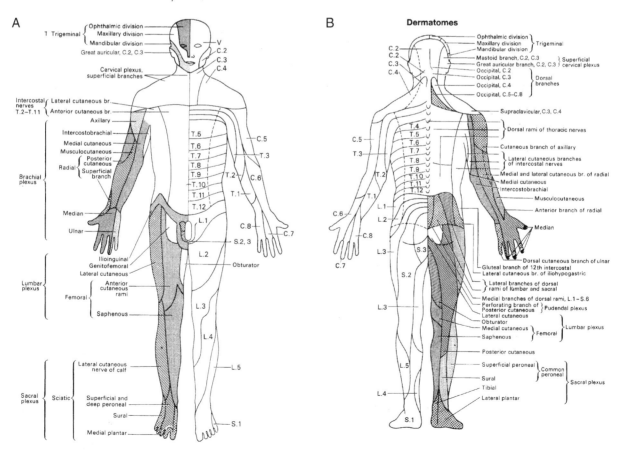

the epidural space. In SCS, the task at hand is to stimulate the nerves that will provide pain relief and avoid the nerves that will produce uncomfortable sensory or motor effects.

Like the sensory cortex in the brain, the DC is organized somatotopically; in the DC, the lateral fibers represent more rostral dermatomes (owing to their more recent entry from their respective DR fibers), and medial fibers innervate more caudal structures.[8–11,13] Thus, at any given level, the DC contains information for all the dermatomes below that level. For this reason the lower extremities can, in some circumstances, be stimulated with a cervical lead (Fig. 5.4).

The nerve root fibers actually enter the cord several segments higher up than their corresponding vertebral entry-point level. Thus, to obtain a paresthesia in a desired dermatome, it is necessary to stimulate the DC several segments cephalad to the homonymous vertebral level. For example, to stimulate the L3 to L5 dermatomes of the leg, the electrodes would be placed between T9 and T11. Understanding DC organization is important when stimulation of the low back is desired. A number of factors underlie the relative difficulty of stimulating the low back, including cord diameter, CSF thickness, and topographic organization of nerve fibers. Stimulating the low back, usually at dermatomes between L2 and L5, is most often accomplished by placing the lead tips at the midline of T8 to T9. Optimal outcomes are well served by systems able to effectively direct current since the area of the DC that when stimulated produces precise dermatomal coverage—known as the *sweet spot*—can occupy a relatively small area, particularly in low back stimulation.

Frequency, Amplitude, and Pulse Width

Only three variables can be manipulated on any single electrode/contact: frequency, amplitude, and pulse width (PW).

Figure 5.4 Somatotopic representation of the dermatomes in the dorsal columns of the T11 spinal segment. Reprinted from Feirabend HK, Choufoer H, Ploeger S, et al. Morphometry of human superficial dorsal and dorsolateral column fibres: significance to spinal cord stimulation. *Brain* 2002 May;125(Pt 5):1137–49, with permission from Oxford University Press.

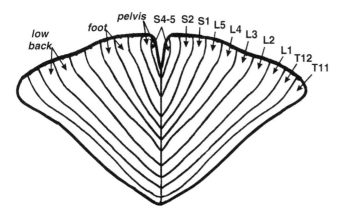

To obtain a paresthesia that roughly overlaps the area of pain, the first step is to select the electrode polarity (i.e., anode, cathode, off) for all implanted contacts; this process "shapes" the electric field surrounding the nerve. Once the paresthesia is in the right area, the amplitude, PW, and frequency are then fine-tuned.

Amplitude (Current/Voltage)

Amplitude affects the intensity and breadth of the paresthesia. It is similar to turning up the volume knob on a sound amplifier. Increasing the amplitude increases the area of capture in the spinal cord, as the expanding electric field recruits more nerves at farther distances from the contacts (see Fig. 5.2).

Increasing amplitude ultimately results in discomfort. Identifying the effective amplitude range for stimulation is accomplished by gradually increasing the stimulation from zero until the patient first reports paresthesia. This is the sensory perception threshold. Increasing further until stimulation is uncomfortable defines the upper limit of stimulation amplitude. The difference in amplitude between these two points is the usage range for stimulation and is often referred to as the *comfort zone*. Ideally, the ratio of the maximum comfortable threshold to the perception threshold is no less than 1.4 to 1.5.[13]

Pulse Width (Microseconds)

The PW is the duration of a single stimulation pulse. Typical clinically used PW ranges from 175 to 600 microseconds (microsecond = one millionth of a second). A stimulus must be of adequate intensity and duration to reach depolarization threshold and generate an action potential in a nerve. The lower the intensity of the stimulus, the longer the stimulus duration must be to evoke a response. The pulse charge or "packet of energy" required to depolarize a nerve is therefore a function of both the amplitude and the PW. Graphs illustrating this relationship are called *strength–duration curves* (Fig. 5.5). Examining strength–duration curves for large and small fibers can help to explain the value of wider PW.[14]

Strength–duration curves for different fiber diameters show three relevant phenomena:

1. Smaller nerve fibers have higher thresholds to depolarization.
2. Higher PW reduces the difference in amplitude needed to stimulate large- and small-diameter nerves.[15]
3. Smaller amplitudes of stimulation at longer PW settings are usually better tolerated by patients.[16,17]

In SCS, increasing PW does not simply increase the size of the stimulation field but actually increases nerve fiber recruitment of both small and large fibers within the stimulation field. When PW is relatively narrow, large fibers are depolarized at lower amplitudes than small fibers. Large fibers will be primarily activated when the PW is narrow. This may yield broad recruitment of large fibers but may not thoroughly recruit the nearby small fibers and may actually promote

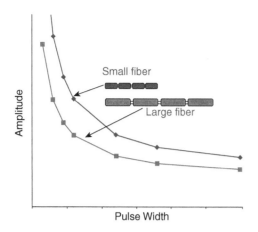

Figure 5.5 Strength–duration curve for large- and small-diameter fibers. Reprinted with permission from Boston Scientific.

recruitment of distal DR fibers.[17] In contrast, when using a wider PW, the stimulation amplitude required to achieve an adequate paresthesia is less and there is more thorough recruitment of both small and large fibers in the nearby DC. Because medial DC fibers tend to be smaller,[18] increasing the PW may actually steer the effective field toward more midline fibers.[17] It is common to start with a PW of 250 microseconds and gradually increase it, depending on the patient's response. One study has shown that a significant number of patients use a PW as high as 1,000 microseconds.[19]

Frequency (Hertz)

The frequency (number of pulses per second) is most often adjusted so that the stimulation sensation is comfortable to the patient. The frequency will influence the quality of the paresthesia (tingling) but is unlikely to affect the location. The initial settings for patients with low back and leg pain usually range from 40 to 70 Hz.[20] Patients with complex regional pain syndrome tend toward higher frequencies, ranging from 80 to 250 Hz.[21]

Single Versus Dual Leads

The decision whether to place one or two leads depends on both the pain condition that is being treated and physician preference. At the inception of percutaneous SCS, a single lead with four electrodes was positioned at various mediolateral points in the epidural space, depending on pain location. If the patient had unilateral extremity pain, the lead was placed a few millimeters off the midline ipsilateral to the painful extremity. If the patient had bilateral extremity pain, which is commonly seen, placement of a single midline lead was attempted in hopes that bilateral stimulation would result in balanced paresthesias in both extremities and that the lead would not migrate laterally, resulting in loss of bilateral stimulation. Unfortunately, lead migration was and continues to be the most common equipment-related complication.[22] With the

development of systems that can deliver stimulation to two leads, many implanters now routinely place dual leads, even for unilateral extremity pain, for the following reasons: (1) In the event of lateral lead migration, stimulation can be electronically transferred horizontally (either medially or laterally) between the two leads to recapture the sweet spot, (2) in patients with bilateral extremity pain, placing each lead slightly off the midline greatly facilitates the perception of stimulation evenly felt in both extremities, and (3) although numerous studies have shown that a single midline lead is best and most efficient in capturing low back pain, any lateral micromigration may result in loss of low back stimulation.[23–25]

As has been shown in mathematical computer modeling studies, two leads placed next to each other, straddling the physiologic midline, can be programmed to "crosstalk" (i.e., superimpose the capture fields and achieve ample penetration into the midline of the DC). The advantage is that the leads can be reprogrammed if lateral micromigration occurs in order to recapture the midline stimulation. No one would condone sloppy lead placement, but placing two leads can offer added benefits in the long run because of the ability, if needed, to correct for lead migration electronically rather than surgically revising and moving the lead back to the specific location over the DC fibers to be stimulated.

Contact Combinations

The terms *monopole, bipole, guarded cathode (tripole), transverse tripole,* and *complex cathode* define the basic geometric distribution of polarity among implanted contacts. However, since each type of contact combination can have different intended clinical effects, it is worthwhile to examine each of these terms separately.

Monopolar Stimulation

Monopolar stimulation is the simplest arrangement, involving an active cathode on the lead and a distant battery case designated as the anode (Fig. 5.6).

Figure 5.6 Monopole stimulation. Reprinted with permission from Boston Scientific.

Monopole Stimulation

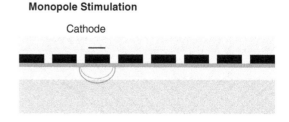

Nerves within range of the cathode will be depolarized and generate an action potential.[26] Remember that cylindrical cathodes, as found on percutaneous leads, create a grossly spherical stimulation field 360 degrees around the cathode.[27] Higher amplitudes result in a greater, generally symmetrical radius of depolarization around the cathode. If the cathode is not directly over the target, a paresthesia will be felt in the wrong location. The anode is remote and does not influence the stimulation pattern.

Bipolar Stimulation

A bipole is created when a single anode and a single cathode are placed next to each other, usually on the same lead, in the epidural space. Because the anode tends to hyperpolarize nerves, the stimulation field will be "pushed away" from the anode toward the cathode, thus moving the field in one direction or another (Fig. 5.7).

Bipoles can be set up vertically with the anode and cathode on the same lead or transversely with the cathode on one lead and the anode lateral to it on a different lead. A transverse bipole would allow the stimulation field to be pushed medio-laterally.[24]

Tripolar Stimulation

Tripolar stimulation is achieved when an anode is placed on both sides of a cathode. This tends to focus the field directly under the cathode because the anodes are effectively "squeezing" the field on either side. The tripole is also called a guarded cathode or guarded tripole (Fig. 5.8).

It is worth noting several facts about tripolar combinations. First, in an important retrospective review, longitudinal guarded cathodes were shown to be chosen by patients significantly more often than other forms of contact combination,[20] suggesting that they have clinical value. However, the implementation of a guarded cathode combination in a single-source stimulator is challenged by differential anode impedances. In such systems, the distribution of anodic current is determined

Figure 5.7 Simple bipole. Reprinted with permission from Boston Scientific.

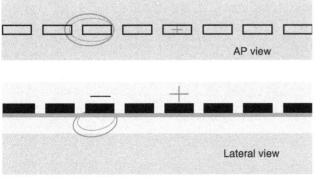

Simple Bipole

AP view

Lateral view

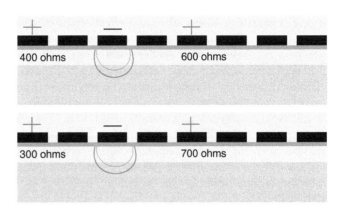

400 ohms   600 ohms

300 ohms   700 ohms

Figure 5.8 Guarded cathode combinations in a single-source stimulator, as influenced by impedance. In a single-source guarded cathode combination, the anodic current from each anode is inversely proportional to the impedance at that contact. Thus, there is less anodic current sourced at the 600-Ohm and 700-Ohm contacts shown, which leads to less hyperpolarization near those contacts than at the 400-Ohm and 300-Ohm contacts respectively. This means the stimulation field will be pushed toward the higher-impedance anodes. These effects will not occur in stimulators that use a current source for each contact. Reprinted with permission from Boston Scientific.

by the impedances on each contact. As can be seen in Figure 5.8, if the impedance of one of the anodic contacts grows progressively larger than the other anodic contact over time, less anodic current will travel through that higher-impedance contact. Less anodic current will lead to less relative hyperpolarization near the higher-impedance contact, and thus the field may theoretically shift. Finally, it is a mistake to assume that even if impedances are equal at all anodes, surrounding the cathode with anodes provides "more shielding." In the guarded cathode combination, the surrounding anodes are only half as strong as those in a bipole. So, while the addition of an anode to a bipole to form a guarded cathode can add some geometric control to the location of stimulation, the "squeezing" of the field becomes less strong with every added anode.

The guarded cathode can be useful in areas in which the sweet spot is narrow and stimulation outside the sweet spot results in stimulation of unwanted structures.[24] Recently, transverse tripoles have been described in which three parallel leads are placed in the dorsal epidural space, with the two lateral leads functioning as anodes and the center lead being the cathode.[28] This may be useful for focusing stimulation on the midline when low back stimulation is desired. New paddle designs incorporating a transverse tripole are being investigated to determine whether they can improve midline stimulation necessary for effective low back stimulation.

Dual or Complex Cathodes, Current Steering, and Interleaving

There are situations in which the desired target of DC lies between two electrodes/contacts. In systems with closely spaced contacts that allow current to be directed, the current can be fractionally divided in small increments (e.g., resolution = 0.1 mA) between two cathodes to move the stimulation field until it precisely covers the desired target. Such "fractionalization" extends the concept of a contact combination from a fixed distribution of polarities to a near-continuum of fractional field shapes. When these field shapes are changed in real time (i.e., when the stimulation amplitude is not reduced to zero before changing the current on a contact), it becomes a process called *current steering*. When programming using cathodic current steering, a single cathode is chosen as a starting point, and the amplitude on that contact is increased until the stimulation is suprathreshold and a comfortable paresthesia is felt. The current steering process occurs by redistributing small fractions of the total delivered current from the original cathode contact to the adjacent cathode contact in an incremental fashion. When this is done using simultaneously delivered pulses and close contact spacing, the stimulation field gradually shifts from underneath the original cathode to the region between the contacts and finally ends up focused under the adjacent contact. An analogy to the steering process might be the sweeping of a searchlight across the sky. Current steering then allows the cathodic field to be moved incrementally down the lead to map the area within reach of the electrodes. Other systems employ a programming methodology known as interleaving (see below) to fine-tune paresthesia location.[29]

The programming unit with some of the newer systems has its own algorithm for electronically "trolling" down the lead(s) using combinations of anodes and cathodes, making it easy to rapidly cycle through hundreds of combinations in a short time.[30] If the patient reports that the area of paresthesia does not correspond with the distribution of pain, moving the cathode between different combinations of electrodes and varying the PW or amplitude is attempted first. If unsuccessful, the lead itself may need to be repositioned.

Electrode Spacing

Reducing the space between electrodes has been shown to improve the ability to steer current and target specific regions of the DC fibers.[31] Closely spaced contacts eliminate gaps in activation regions of the DC that may be present when using leads with widely spaced contacts. Additionally, closely spaced contacts allow for more even incremental shifting, with greater field-shift resolution of the electric field using current steering.[31] One potential disadvantage to tightly spacing leads is that since the number of contacts per lead is currently limited, the length of the active (programmable) portion of the lead (the distance between the first and last contact) is reduced. This can be important when it is necessary to stimulate over more than one vertebral segment (Fig. 5.9).

Pulse Generators

Electrical Stimulation Technology

Implantable electrical stimulation systems must be designed to safely deliver current over a long duration of implant. An improperly designed system can potentially lead to tissue damage or damage to the electrodes. Similar to electroplating, corrosion can occur at the anode if the potential exceeds the threshold at which oxidation occurs. It has been shown that uncontrolled tissue stimulation can cause tissue damage. In uncontrolled systems, disruption of biologic processes occurs as a result of net charge transfer from the stimulation system to the surrounding biologic environment. The tissue damage demonstrated in animal models was the result of toxic electrochemical reactions that occur at the surface of the electrodes that the surrounding tissue cannot buffer. Additionally, animal studies have suggested that overstimulation can affect neural systems. Mass action theory suggests that this phenomenon occurs when multiple neurons fire, resulting in local changes in pH and electrolyte balance, as well as excessive release of excitatory amino acids such as glutamate.

To prevent these damaging phenomena, all modern pulse generators use a biphasic form of stimulation that recovers injected charge between pulses to prevent charge imbalance from building up. Biphasic pulses return the electrode back to a steady-state charge after each stimulation pulse and recovery. Using only unidirectional monophasic pulsing results in current moving only toward the cathode, and a charge builds up on the contacts, causing the electrode to break down over time. Damage to surrounding tissue results from pH changes and free radical generation.

Often, a short delay is placed between the first stimulating phase and the following recovery phase (in which current is

Figure 5.9 SCS leads.

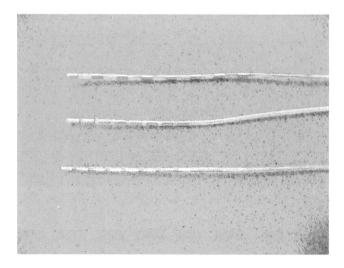

injected backward through the cathode to neutralize any charge buildup). A short amount of time between the two phases (interphase) improves activation of the targeted nerves.[32]

The concept seems simple enough, but the electrochemical analysis and programming used to derive the correct interphase delay and charge to be injected between pulses to prevent charge imbalance without creating a damaging overpotential of the electrode is complex and beyond the scope of this text.

Power Sources: Rechargeable, Nonrechargeable, and Radiofrequency

Three types of pulse generator power sources are available: radiofrequency (RF), nonrechargeable batteries (a.k.a. primary cell), and rechargeable batteries.

RF units are implanted receivers that obtain power from an external source taped over the skin above the receiver. These were the first fully implantable devices to be used for SCS and were the only units available in the 1970s. With an RF unit, no battery replacement surgery is ever required because the battery is external; however, the patient must wear an antenna taped to the skin over the receiver for the system to function. This system is undesirable for many patients because the external battery can interfere with normal activities and the tape required to secure the antenna can cause chronic skin irritation. Because functional improvement is a primary goal, a device that interferes with normal functioning, such as sleeping, showering, or swimming, may be less than optimal for many patients. Although still available, with the development of rechargeable batteries, RF systems are now used less frequently.

Nonrechargeable IPGs containing primary cell lithium and silver-vanadium-oxide batteries were introduced in 1980 and were developed based on pacemaker technology. The RF unit and the primary cell battery were the only choices available for more than 20 years. There were tradeoffs in choosing between these two types of generators. Depending on power usage, most patients would require a primary cell IPG replacement every 3 to 4 years, although some patients would require yearly replacement. Even though an RF stimulator had no power constraints because the battery was external, their multiple inconveniences led many patients to endure frequent battery exchanges rather than accept an RF system.

Rechargeable lithium-ion batteries became available for SCS in 2004. Rechargeable batteries offer a renewable power source and are therefore capable of supplying higher output for a greater number of leads and contacts while simultaneously maintaining higher amplitudes, frequencies, and PWs. Rechargeable battery technology also maintains longer intervals between battery replacement. However, all implanted batteries, rechargeable or nonrechargeable, will inevitably wear out and need to be replaced.

Currently available rechargeable batteries are specified to last up to 9 years, although improvements in battery technology should extend these lifetimes. For optimal recharging to occur, all batteries are implanted to a maximum depth of 2 to 2.5 cm, depending on the manufacturer's specifications (although these recommended depths are in keeping with previous primary-cell and RF implant recommendations).

Pacemakers and Implanted Pulse Generators: Are They Compatible?

There is a single 1993 case report in the medical literature documenting reported interference between a unipolar pacemaker and a unipolar SCS implant. The same author in 1998 subsequently published a case report demonstrating the safe use of a dual-pacing, dual-sensing, dual-mode pacemaker in a patient with implanted quadripolar SCS electrodes. A recent poster session presented five patients with both SCS and pacemakers who experienced no electrical interference between the two units. We recommend consulting the manufacturers of both companies before considering patients with pacemakers for SCS.[33,34]

Current Versus Voltage Control

IPGs differ in their delivery of energy to electrodes. Energy can be delivered to the electrodes by controlling either voltage or current. From an electrophysiologic standpoint, it is the amount of current flow to the spinal cord neurons that determines the region of fibers to be stimulated. Some systems are able to control exactly how much energy is delivered to each electrode on a lead, whereas others simply deliver energy to the lead and divide it between selected electrodes, the division of energy being determined by the impedance at each contact. In voltage-controlled systems, pulse amplitude is defined in terms of a fixed voltage. Changes in impedance will result in changes in total current flow and in turn change the intensity of stimulation perceived. Current-controlled systems deliver constant-current pulses to the electrodes regardless of the total impedance. This has both short- and long-term ramifications. First, it has been shown that impedance increases during the delivery of a single pulse from the generator.[35] In voltage-controlled systems, this results in a rapid decrease in delivered current from the beginning to the end of the pulse (i.e., "tilted" current pulses), which can become significant when longer pulse durations are used. Second, variable impedances are seen at each contact, which can change unpredictably over time.[30] It is believed that disproportionate amounts of fibrotic tissue form around each contact, with the amount of fibrosis per contact changing over time. Systems with the ability to independently program individual contacts or with complex interleaving programming capability can often overcome the effects of variable fibrosis formation, potentially reducing the incidence of discordant paresthesia.[36]

Independently Controlled Current Delivery

There is currently one SCS system available that uses independent current delivery to each contact. The analogy of the household water faucet is useful in considering independent contact programming. Voltage is analogous to water pressure at the source, current is analogous to water flowing out of the end of the faucet, and resistance is the diameter of the pipe between the source and the faucet. Typically, a water faucet has its own control, allowing one to individually adjust each faucet, akin to controlling the resistance. If there is a decrease in water pressure to the house, the faucet can be opened up further to maintain the same output. This can be done for each faucet. Multiple activities can be performed at once (e.g., showering, washing clothes, doing the dishes), and the water output can be adjusted specifically for each activity. This is analogous to individual current control at each contact.

Interleaved Pulses in Nonindependently Controlled Current/Voltage Delivery Systems

Interleaving is another means of controlling paresthesia location. Modern pulse generators have increased programming capabilities that allow multiple channels to be run concurrently, using pulse interleaving. Interleaved stimulation is defined as "pulse-to-pulse variation in pulse amplitude, pulse width, and contact assignment."[29] As shown in Figure 5.10, two interleaved channels, A and B, can be run such that their

pulses alternate in time. The clinical effect of such interleaving is that some neurons will feel only the effect of channel A (left non-dashed circle), other neurons will feel only the effect of channel B (right non-dashed circle), while other neurons will feel the effect of both channels (intersection of both non-dashed circles). Since the stimulation rates used in interleaving tend to be those used for single-channel stimulation (e.g., 40 to 70 Hz), and the interpulse interval between the two interleaved channels is typically several milliseconds, the expected effect of the A+B neurons in the intersection region would be a higher rate of action potential generation rather than any greater recruitment than that due to A alone or B alone. Most often, interleaving is used to allow independent control of stimulated body regions. This is possible because the interleaving of pulses, while likely recruiting no more fibers in the spinal cord, results in paresthesias that are perceived concurrently by the patient—that is, if channel A recruits the left foot and channel B recruits the left knee, the patient perceives both the left foot and knee as "on at the same time." This allows the channels to be separately controlled by the patient: the patient may increase the paresthesia intensity on the foot (channel A amplitude increased) without affecting the paresthesia on the knee (channel B unchanged).[29,37]

REFERENCES

1. North RB, Lanning A, Hessels R, et al. Spinal cord stimulation with percutaneous and plate electrodes: side effects and quantitative comparisons. *Neurosurg Focus* 1997;2(1:3):1–5.
2. North RB, Kidd DH, Olin J, et al. Spinal cord stimulation electrode design: prospective, controlled trial comparing percutaneous and laminectomy electrodes—Part I: technical outcomes. *Neurosurgery* 2002;51(2):381–90.
3. North RB, Kidd DH, Petrucci L, et al. Spinal cord stimulation electrode design: a prospective, randomized, controlled trial comparing percutaneous with laminectomy electrodes—Part II: clinical outcomes. *Neurosurgery* 2005;57(5):990–5.
4. Oakley et al. *Variability of contact impedance over time in SCS.* American Society of Stereotactic and Functional Neurosurgery Biennial Meeting: Neuromodulation, Defining the Future, Oct. 1–3, 2004.
5. Alò K, Varga C, Krames E, et al. Factors affecting impedance of percutaneous leads in spinal cord stimulation. *Neuromodulation* 2006;9(2):128–35.
6. Barolat G. Experience with 509 plate electrodes implanted epidurally from C1 to L1. *Stereotact Funct Neurosurg* 1993;61(2):60–79.
7. Barolat G, Schwartzman R, Woo R. Epidural spinal cord stimulation in the management of reflex sympathetic dystrophy. *Stereotact Funct Neurosurg* 1989;53(1):29–39.
8. Holsheimer J, Barolat G, Struijk JJ, He J. Significance of the spinal cord position in spinal cord stimulation. *Acta Neurochir Suppl* 1995;64:119–24.
9. Holsheimer J, Khan YN, Raza SS, et al. Effects of electrode positioning on perception threshold and paresthesia coverage in spinal cord stimulation. *Neuromodulation* 2007;10(1):34–41.
10. Holsheimer J, Struijk JJ. How do geometric factors influence epidural spinal cord stimulation? A quantitative analysis by computer modeling. *Stereotact Funct Neurosurg* 1991;56(4):234–49.

Figure 5.10 Intersecting paresthesia. When intersecting paresthesia areas A and B overlap pain, the area of intersection, A + B, is exposed to frequency doubling. Reprinted with permission from North RB, Kidd DH, Olin J, Sieracki JM, Boulay M. Spinal cord stimulation with interleaved pulses: a randomized, controlled trial. *Neuromodulation* 2007;10(4):349–57 with permission from Wiley Publishing.

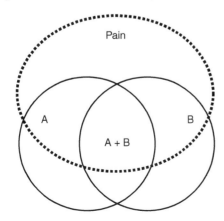

11. Holsheimer J, Wesselink WA. Optimum electrode geometry for spinal cord stimulation: the narrow bipole and tripole. *Med Biol Eng Comput* 1997;35(5):493–7.

12. Ko H-Y, Park JH, Shin YB, et al. Gross quantitative measurements of spinal cord segments in humans. *Spinal Cord* 2004;42:35–40.

13. He J, Barolat G, Holsheimer J, et al. Perception threshold and electrode position for spinal cord stimulation. *Pain* 1994;59(1):55–63.

14. Merrill DR, Bikson M, Jefferys JG. Electrical stimulation of excitable tissue: design of efficacious and safe protocols. *J Neurosci Methods* 2005;141:171–98.

15. Mortimer JT, Bhadra N. Peripheral nerve and muscle stimulation. In: Horch KW, Dhillon GS, eds. *Neuroprosthetics: theory and practice*. New Jersey: World Scientific Publishing, 2004.

16. Jobling DT, Tallis RC, Illis LS. Electronic aspects of spinal-cord stimulation in multiple sclerosis. *Med Biol Eng Comput* 1980;18(1):48–56.

17. Yearwood TL. Neuropathic extremity pain and spinal cord stimulation. *Pain Med* 2006;7(1):S97–S102.

18. Feirabend HK, Choufoer H, Ploeger S, et al. Morphometry of human superficial dorsal and dorsolateral column fibres: significance to spinal cord stimulation. *Brain* 2002;125:1137–49.

19. Gould B, Dradley K. *Pulse width programming in spinal cord stimulators*. Poster, American Academy of Pain Medicine 22nd Annual Meeting, February 2006, San Diego.

20. North RB, Kidd DH, Zahurak M, et al. Spinal cord stimulation for chronic, intractable pain: experience over two decades. *Neurosurgery* 1993;32(3):384–94.

21. Bennett DS, Aló KM, Oakley J, et al. Spinal cord stimulation for complex regional pain syndrome I (RSD). A retrospective multicenter experience from 1995–1998 of 101 patients. *Neuromodulation* 1999;2(3):202–10.

22. Cameron T. Safety and efficacy of spinal cord stimulation for the treatment of chronic pain: a 20-year literature review. *J Neurosurg* 2004;100(3):254–67.

23. North RB, Kidd DA, Olin J, et al. Spinal cord stimulation for axial low back pain: a prospective controlled trial comparing 16-contact insulated electrodes with 4-contact percutaneous electrodes. *Neuromodulation* 2006;0(1):56–67.

24. Wesselink WA, Holsheimer J, King GW, et al. Quantitative aspects of the clinical performance of transverse tripolar spinal cord stimulation. *Neuromodulation* 1999;2(1):5–14.

25. Barolat G, Oakley JC, Law JD, et al. Epidural spinal cord stimulation with a multiple electrode paddle lead is effective in treating intractable low back pain. *Neuromodulation* 2001;4(2):59–66.

26. Ranck JB Jr. Which elements are excited in electrical stimulation of mammalian central nervous system: a review. *Brain Res* 1975;98(3):417–40.

27. Dimitrejvic MR, Gregoric MR, Sherwood AM, et al. Reflex responses of paraspinal muscles to tapping. *J Neurol Neurosurg Psych* 1980;43(12):1112–8.

28. Holsheimer J, Wesselink WA. Effect of anode-cathode configuration on paresthesia coverage in spinal cord stimulation. *Neurosurgery* 1997;41:654–60.

29. North RB, Kidd DH, Olin J, et al. Spinal cord stimulation with interleaved pulses: a randomized, controlled trial. *Neuromodulation* 2007;10(4):349–57.

30. Oakley J, Varga C, Krames E, et al. Real-time paresthesia steering using continuous electric field adjustment. Part I: Intraoperative performance. *Neuromodulation* 2004;7(3):157–67.

31. Manola L, Holsheimer J, Veltink P, et al. Anodal vs. cathodal stimulation of motor cortex: a modeling study. *Clin Neurophysiol* 2007;118(2):464–74.

32. Bonner M, Mortimer JT, Daroux M. Engineering in Medicine and Biology Society. Effect of pulsewidth and delay on stimulating electrode charge injection in-vitro. *Proc 12th Ann Int Conf IEEE* 1990;1–4:1482–3.

33. Krakovsky AA. *Cardiac pacemaker and spinal cord stimulator: do they interfere?* American Academy of Pain Medicine Poster Session, Poster No. 104, February 2006.

34. Romano M, Brusa S, Grieco A, et al. Efficacy and safety of permanent cardiac DDD pacing with contemporaneous double spinal cord stimulation. *Pacing Clin Electrophysiol* 1998;21:465–7.

35. Butson C, McIntyre C. Differences among implanted pulse generator waveforms cause variations in the neural response to deep brain stimulation. *Clin Neurophysiol* 2007;118(8):1889–94.

36. Aló KM, Holsheimer J. New trends in neuromodulation for the management of neuropathic pain. *Neurosurgery* 2002;50(4):690–704.

37. Aló KM, Yland MI, Redko V, et al. Multiple program spinal cord stimulation in the treatment of chronic pain: follow-up of multiple program SCS. *Neuromodulation* 1999;2(4):266–72.

Further Reading

Aló KM, Redko V, Charnov J. Four-year follow-up of dual electrode spinal cord stimulation for chronic pain. *Neuromodulation* 2002;5(2):79–99.

Aló KM, Yland MJ, Kramer DL, et al. Computer assisted and patient interactive programming of dual electrode spinal cord stimulation in the treatment of chronic pain. *Neuromodulation* 1998;1(1):30–45.

Barolat G, Massaro F, He J, et al. Mapping of sensory responses to epidural stimulation of the intraspinal neural structures in man. *J Neurosurg* 1993;78(2):233–9.

Blond S, Armignies P, Parker F, et al. Chronic sciatalgia caused by sensitive deafferentiation following surgery for lumbar disk hernia: clinical and therapeutic aspects. Apropos of 110 patients [in French]. *Neurochirurgie* 1991;37(2):86–95.

Broseta J, Roldan P, Gonzalez-Darder J, et al. Chronic epidural dorsal column stimulation in the treatment of causalgic pain. *Appl Neurophysiol* 1982;45:190–4.

Burchiel KJ, Anderson VC, Brown FD, et al. Prospective, multicenter study of spinal cord stimulation for relief of chronic back and extremity pain. *Spine* 1996;21(23):2786–94.

De Andres J, Quiroz C, Villanueva V, et al. Patient satisfaction with spinal cord stimulation for failed back surgery syndrome [in Spanish]. *Rev Esp Anestesiol Reanim* 2007;54(1):17–22.

de la Porte C, Siegfried J. Lumbosacral spinal fibrosis (spinal arachnoiditis). Its diagnosis and treatment by spinal cord stimulation. *Spine* 1983;8(6):593–603.

Erickson DL. Percutaneous trial of stimulation for patient selection for implantable stimulating devices. *J Neurosurg* 1975;34:440–4.

Forouzanfar T, Kemler MA, Weber WE, et al. Spinal cord stimulation in complex regional pain syndrome: cervical and lumbar devices are comparably effective. *Br J Anaesth* 2004;92(3):348–53.

Heidecke V, Rainov NG, Burkert W. Hardware failures in spinal cord stimulation for failed back surgery syndrome. *Neuromodulation* 2000;3(1):27–30.

Holsheimer J, Nuttin B, King GW, et al. Clinical evaluation of paresthesia steering with a new system for spinal cord stimulation. *Neurosurgery* 1998;42(3):541–7.

Holsheimer J, Struijk JJ. *Effects of electrode geometry and combination on paresthesia coverage and usage range in ESCS*. Proceedings of the Second Congress of the International Neuromodulation Society, Göteborg, Sweden, 1994.

Hoppenstein R. Electrical stimulation of the ventral and dorsal columns of the spinal cord for relief of chronic intractable pain: preliminary report. *Surg Neurol* 1975;4(1):187–94.

Hosobuchi Y, Adams JE, Weinstein PR. Preliminary percutaneous dorsal column stimulation prior to permanent implantation. *J Neurosurg* 1972;17:242–5.

Kay AD, McIntyre MD, Macrae WA, et al. Spinal cord stimulation—a long-term evaluation in patients with chronic pain. *Br J Neurosurg* 2001;15(4):335–41.

Krainick JU, Thoden U, Riechert T. Spinal cord stimulation in post-amputation pain. *Surg Neurol* 1975;4(1):167–70.

Kumar A, Felderhof C, Eljamel MS. Spinal cord stimulation for the treatment of refractory unilateral limb pain syndromes. *Stereotact Funct Neurosurg* 2003;81(1–4):70–4.

Kumar K, Hunter G, Demeria D. Spinal cord stimulation in treatment of chronic benign pain: challenges in treatment planning and present status, a 22-year experience. *Neurosurgery* 2006; 58(3):481–96.

Kumar K, Malik S, Demeria D. Treatment of chronic pain with spinal cord stimulation versus alternative therapies: cost-effectiveness analysis. *Neurosurgery* 2002;51(1):106–15.

Kumar K, Nath TK, Toth C. Spinal cord stimulation is effective in the management of reflex sympathetic dystrophy. *Neurosurgery* 1997;40(3):503–8.

Kumar K, Nath R, Wyant GM. Treatment of chronic pain by epidural spinal cord stimulation: a 10-year experience. *J Neurosurg* 1991; 75(3):402–7.

Kumar K, Toth C. The role of spinal cord stimulation in the treatment of chronic pain postlaminectomy. *Curr Pain Headache Rep* 1998;2:85–92.

Kumar K, Toth C, Nath RK, Laing P. Epidural spinal cord stimulation for treatment of chronic pain—some predictors of success. A 15-year experience. *Surg Neurol* 1998;50(2):110–20.

Kumar K, Wilson JR, Taylor RS, et al. Complications of spinal cord stimulation, suggestions to improve outcome, and financial impact. *J Neurosurg Spine* 2006;5(3):191–203.

Lang P. The treatment of chronic pain by epidural spinal cord stimulation—a 15-year follow-up: present status. *Axon* 1997; 71–3.

Leveque JC, Villavicencio AT, Bulsara KR, et al. Spinal cord stimulation for failed back surgery syndrome. *Neuromodulation* 2001; 4(1):1–9.

May MS, Banks C, Thomson SJ. A retrospective, long-term, third-party follow-up of patients considered for spinal cord stimulation. *Neuromodulation* 2002;5(3):137–44.

Meglio M, Cioni B, Rossi GF. Spinal cord stimulation in management of chronic pain. A 9-year experience. *J Neurosurg* 1989;70(4): 519–24.

Meglio M, Cioni B, Visocchi M, et al. Spinal cord stimulation in low back and leg pain. *Stereotact Funct Neurosurg* 1994;62(1-4): 263–6.

North RB, Brigham DD, Khalessi A, et al. Spinal cord stimulator adjustment to maximize implanted battery longevity: a randomized, controlled trial using a computerized, patient-interactive programmer. *Neuromodulation* 2004;7(1):13–25.

North RB, Calkins SK, Campbell DS, et al. Automated, patient-interactive spinal cord stimulator adjustment: a randomized, controlled trial. *Neurosurgery* 2003;52(3):572–9.

North RB, Fischell TA, Long DM. Chronic stimulation via percutaneously inserted epidural electrodes. *Neurosurgery* 1977;1(2):215–8.

North RB, Fischell TA, Long DM. Chronic dorsal column stimulation via percutaneously inserted epidural electrodes: preliminary results in 31 patients. *Appl Neurophysiol* 1977-8;40(2–4):184–91.

North RB, Fowler K, Nigrin DJ, et al. Patient-interactive, computer-controlled neurological stimulation system: clinical efficacy in spinal cord stimulator adjustment. *J Neurosurg* 1992;76(6):967–72.

North RB, Kidd DH, Olin J, et al. Spinal cord stimulation for axial low back pain: a prospective, controlled trial comparing dual with single percutaneous electrodes. *Spine* 2005;30(12):1412–8.

North RB, Nigrin DJ, Fowler KR, et al. Automated "pain drawing" analysis by computer-controlled, patient-interactive neurological stimulation system. *Pain* 1992;50(1):51–7.

North RB, Sieracki JN, Fowler KR, et al. Patient-interactive, microprocessor-controlled neurological stimulation system. *Neuromodulation* 1998;1(4):185–93.

Quigley DG, Arnold J, Eldridge PR, et al. Long-term outcome of spinal cord stimulation and hardware complications. *Stereotact Funct Neurosurg* 2003;81(1–4):50–6.

Racz GB, McCarron RF, Talboys P. Percutaneous dorsal column stimulator for chronic pain control. *Spine* 1989;14(1):1–4.

Rosenow JM, Stanton-Hicks M, Rezai AR, et al. Failure modes of spinal cord stimulation hardware. *J Neurosurg Spine* 2006;5:183–90.

Simpson BA, Bassett G, Davies K, et al. Cervical spinal cord stimulation for pain: a report on 41 patients. *Neuromodulation* 2003; 6(1):20–6.

Sundaraj SR, Johnstone C, Noore F, et al. Spinal cord stimulation: a seven-year audit. *J Clin Neurosci* 2005;12(3):264–70.

Vallejo R, Kramer J, Benyamin R. Neuromodulation of the cervical spinal cord in the treatment of chronic intractable neck and upper extremity pain: a case series and review of the literature. *Pain Physician* 2007;10(2):305–11.

Van Buyten J-P, van Zundert J, Vueghs P, et al. Efficacy of spinal cord stimulation: 10 years of experience in a pain centre in Belgium. *Eur J Pain* 2001;5(3):299–307.

6

Trial of Spinal Cord Stimulation: Basic Considerations

Introduction

Patients must successfully complete a screening trial before being considered as candidates for implantation of a permanent spinal cord stimulation (SCS) system. Such trials can be critically informative and may indicate how comfortable the patient will be with SCS and which lead locations and stimulation settings will be most effective. It is crucial that the technical aspects of the trial be performed optimally because permanent implantation will depend on a successful trial. The goal of the screening trial is lead placement that achieves a paresthesia covering the entire area of pain. Successful topographic coverage of the paresthesia, however, does not ensure clinical success, as some patients in whom complete coverage is achieved still report little or no pain relief. Other patients find early in the trial that they dislike the sensation of the paresthesia altogether. It is therefore necessary to perform a screening trial of sufficient length to forecast long-term efficacy and identify short-term failure, while minimizing infection risk. A trial of 3 to 8 days generally provides sufficient information and is short enough to reduce infection risk.[1,2]

Percutaneous Versus Tunneled Trials

Prior to permanent SCS implantation, a patient may undergo one of two types of trials: a percutaneous (temporary) trial or a tunneled (permanent) trial. A percutaneous trial involves the temporary placement of a disposable trial lead, whereas a tunneled trial involves permanently implanting the trial lead, which eventually will be used for the permanent implant. The decision of whether to undertake a percutaneous or tunneled trial has important procedural implications and must therefore be made in advance of the trial.

In a percutaneous trial, lead implantation can usually be accomplished in an office fluoroscopy suite. The leads are placed percutaneously into the epidural space and are connected to a pulse generator, which is left external to the body. The leads exit through a small puncture wound in the skin: neither a skin incision nor a midline pocket is required to anchor the lead to the paraspinous fascia. The trial typically lasts 3 to 8 days. At the end of the trial, the patient is seen in the office and the temporary leads are removed and discarded. If the trial is successful, permanent surgical implantation is scheduled.

In tunneled trials, lead implantation must be performed in an operating room (OR). The leads are surgically anchored to the paraspinous fascia through a midline incision and are coiled into a midline pocket. Extensions are connected to the leads at the midline and are then tunneled laterally and subcutaneously to prevent contamination of the leads and midline pocket. The lead extensions exit the skin percutaneously and are connected to an external pulse generator. After the trial, the patient returns to the OR where, depending on the success or failure of the trial, the leads are either left in place and attached to a new implanted pulse generator or surgically removed. Obviously, the intent is to use the trial leads for the permanent implant.

Each type of trial has advantages and disadvantages, which are discussed further here.

Advantages of Percutaneous Trials

Percutaneous trials require only needle insertion, eliminating the need for incision and the resultant post-trial scar. Patients tend to be more accepting of this trial because, upon its completion, the leads may be removed and the individual is quickly able to resume previous activities.

The percutaneous trial can be performed in a conventional fluoroscopy suite, whereas a tunneled trial must be performed in an OR, which significantly increases the expense.

There is less pain associated with a percutaneous trial, which allows the patient to be more active and facilitates evaluation of the trial's efficacy. A percutaneous trial may suggest different lead locations for the permanent implant, which can improve efficacy.

If the trial is unsuccessful, the consequences for the patient are less severe. There is less postoperative pain and no surgical incision, which reduces the risk of infection, and the leads can be painlessly removed in the clinic.

Disadvantages of Percutaneous Trials

If it is difficult to position the lead or to obtain adequate stimulation during a percutaneous trial, it may be even more difficult or impossible to do so at the time of permanent implantation. The time between the trial and permanent implantation is longer with percutaneous than with tunneled trials. Finally, the discarded trial leads increase the material cost of permanent implantation.

Advantages of Tunneled Trials

A tunneled trial is the optimal choice if lead placement is anticipated to be difficult. Correct placement can often be the most difficult part of the procedure, and percutaneous trials may often lead to situations where concordant paresthesia cannot be obtained with the permanent implant.

The time between the trial and permanent implantation is shorter with tunneled trials than with percutaneous trials because the patient goes directly to permanent implantation at the end of the trial.

The trial leads become part of the permanent implantation, eliminating the cost of permanent leads and reducing the surgical time required for permanent implantation. However, equipment cost savings may not offset the additional cost incurred in OR charges.

Disadvantages of Tunneled Trials

Tunneled leads must be implanted in the OR, and a subsequent OR appointment must be scheduled for lead removal if the trial is not successful, resulting in significantly increased cost.

Regardless of success, a tunneled trial always involves a midline incision and a post-trial scar. These patients may feel pressured to proceed with the permanent system, even if it does not optimally alleviate pain, because they have already invested significant time and effort (i.e., "I've come this far, I might as well go ahead").

The risk of infection may be higher with tunneled leads because the midline incision must be reopened, potentially allowing bacteria to enter the pocket along the extension tunnel, although recent data regarding tunneled epidural infusions and low infection rates appear to largely negate this argument.[3]

If the trial suggests revising the lead location, repositioning can potentially be difficult and time-consuming.

A tunneled trial is more painful, which may make early evaluation of efficacy ambiguous because the patient is less active, taking more medications for acute pain, or both.

It is our observation and opinion that the majority of trials performed in the United States are percutaneous and not tunneled, although there is support in the literature for using a tunneled trial lead for the permanent implantation.[4] According to some experts, permanent trials appear to be more commonly performed in Europe and Australia, perhaps due to their socialized medical systems and the hospital DRG requirements. Having said this, we prefer a percutaneous trial.

General Information About Percutaneous Trials

Equipment

The trial SCS system consists of three parts: the lead that will be implanted in the epidural space, the external pulse generator, and optional extension wires that connect the lead to the pulse generator. Also required for SCS trials are programming units through which stimulation variables are adjusted. Implantation kits containing the leads, equipment, and other tools necessary to implant the SCS system are available from manufacturers.

Epidural leads, which have stimulating electrodes at the distal end and a connector at the proximal end, can be either percutaneous or surgical. Percutaneous leads are cylindrical catheters with sequentially spaced electrodes at the distal end of the catheter that vary in the number of electrodes and spacing between the electrodes depending on the manufacturer. The percutaneous electrode design allows current to flow symmetrically, creating 360-degree stimulation. Cylindrical spacers separate each electrode on the catheter. Percutaneous leads are placed through a Tuohy needle with a large flat bevel and can be used for percutaneous trials, tunneled trials, or permanent implantation. It is common to place more than one lead in order to provide adequate stimulation and provide redundancy in the event of minor lead migration.

Surgical paddle leads are placed via a surgical laminotomy and have larger, flatter, paddle-shaped electrode surfaces, although new paddle leads designs are being tested that are only slightly wider than percutaneous leads. Surgical paddle leads are designed to reduce migration and to provide unidirectional stimulation over a large area. Paddle leads are usually placed by neurosurgeons or orthopaedic spine surgeons and are not covered further here.

Pulse generators, or neurostimulators, provide the electrical power for stimulation as well as the programmable electronics. The totally implanted pulse generator contains a lithium battery and is self-contained. The advent of rechargeable pulse generators has allowed for more liberal power consumption. Radiofrequency pulse generators equipped with a receiver and an antenna in order to communicate with an external battery-powered transmitter are falling out of favor.

Extension wires connect the lead to the pulse stimulator. One extension per lead is implanted.

Test screeners are external power sources, typically used by manufacturer's representatives, that attach to lead extensions and allow intraoperative and post-trial implant setup and testing of the SCS system. Manufacturer's representatives are usually available to assist in selecting a combination of anodes and cathodes, amplitude, pulse width, and stimulation frequency that produce a comfortable concordant paresthesia and provide the highest degree of pain relief. At present, most test screeners are integrated into a laptop computer or a PDA device. Programmers are used for programming totally implanted SCS systems and allow stimulation variables to be adjusted using telemetry.

Implant kits generally include a Tuohy needle, SCS lead, guidewire, tunneling tools, anchors, a screening cable, stylets, and a percutaneous extension for trials of SCS. Kits are also available for implanting permanent extension wires and for pulse generators.

Relevant Anatomy of the Epidural Space

A thorough understanding and appreciation of the three-dimensional anatomy of the spine, including bone, vascular structures, epidural space, spinal cord, and other neuronal structures, is indispensable when implanting SCS leads and pulse generators. Because soft tissue structures cannot be seen on fluoroscopy imaging, the location must be inferred from identifiable bony structures (e.g., spinous process, articular processes, pedicles, and lamina).

Three membranes surround the spinal cord: the dura mater, arachnoid mater, and pia mater span from outermost to innermost (Fig. 6.1).

The outermost membrane—the dura mater or theca—is a fibroelastic membrane that extends from the foramen magnum to the second sacral vertebra. It is separated from the arachnoid mater by the subdural space, which contains only small amounts of serous fluid (Table 6.1). This space is not intentionally used in anesthesia.

Figure 6.1 Cross-sectional anatomy of spinal cord. Reprinted with permission from A.D.A.M Health Solutions, Inc.

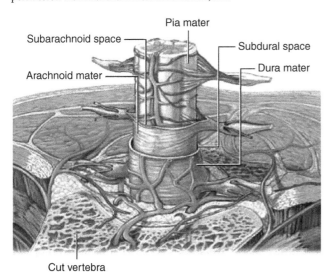

Pia mater
Subarachnoid space
Subdural space
Dura mater
Arachnoid mater
Cut vertebra

The epidural space lies external to, and surrounds, the dura mater. Just ventral to the intralaminar area, the epidural space is bounded posteriorly by the ligamentum flavum, anteriorly by the dura, and laterally by the vertebral pedicles and intervertebral foramina. It is composed of nerve roots, lymphatics, blood vessels, and fatty areolar tissue. The epidural fat is fairly vascular and appears to serve as a shock absorber to protect the contents of the epidural space. Epidural veins are primarily located anterolaterally in the epidural space. Epidural arteries are present, with the most significant anastomoses lying in the lateral epidural space. Increased fat stores elsewhere in the body are associated with increased epidural fat. The epidural space extends from the foramen magnum to the sacral hiatus (see Table 6.1).

The cervical epidural space extends from the dura of the foramen magnum to the inferior border of C7. The thoracic epidural space begins at C7 and extends to the upper margin of the L1 vertebra. The lumbosacral epidural space extends from the upper margin of the L1 vertebra inferiorly to the sacrococcygeal ligament.

The distance between the ligamentum flavum and the dura varies with location in the spinal column. The greatest distance is at L2, where, in adults, it measures 5 to 6 mm. In the thoracic spine the distance is approximately 3 to 4 mm. At C7 the distance is reduced to 1.5 to 2 mm because of the enlargement of the cord at that level. The epidural space is more segmented and less uniform than once believed. The ligamentum flavum is likewise not uniform along the length of the spine, nor even within the intervertebral space. The ligament is absent entirely at the midline in the upper thoracic spine in a significant percentage of individuals, as explained in the next section.

Lead Locations in the Spine

Although ideal lead positioning may vary significantly from patient to patient, certain patterns frequently recur. Cervical stimulation often involves treating one or both of the upper extremities, especially after unsuccessful cervical surgery or in patients with complex regional pain syndrome. As noted previously, to obtain a paresthesia in a desired dermatome it is necessary to stimulate the dorsal column several segments cephalad to that level. Shoulder stimulation is often obtained with the lead placed slightly off midline between C2 and C4. Upper extremity stimulation can most often be achieved by placing the lead slightly off midline between C3 and C4 and then moving inferiorly as necessary to stimulate more medially in the forearm or hand. Placing two leads, each slightly off the physiologic midline to the right and left between C4 and C6, will often allow for bilateral upper extremity stimulation. In 40% of patients, the anatomic (vertebral) and physiologic (spinal cord) midlines may differ by as much as 2 mm at all spinal cord levels.[5] For this reason, the first lead should always be tested for paresthesia location before the second lead is placed. Lateral fluoroscopy should always be performed to document placement of the leads within the epidural space.[6]

Table 6.1

Layers Between the Skin and the Spinal Cord

Layer	Characteristics	Notes
Skin		
Subcutaneous tissue		
Supraspinous ligament		
Interspinous ligament		
Ligamentum flavum	May not be fused at the midline in the upper thoracic region	Actually two ligaments variably joined at the midline
Epidural space	Thinner at the cervical spine; thicker (5–6 mm at the midline) at the lumbar spine. Contains nerve roots, fat, areolar tissue, lymphatics, blood vessels.	
Dura mater (theca)	Fibroelastic membrane	
Subdural space	Small amounts of serous fluid	Easily perforated by the needle
Arachnoid mater	Delicate membrane	Principal barrier to drugs moving into and out of the cerebral spinal fluid; accounts for 90% of the resistance to drug migration
Subarachnoid space	Contains cerebrospinal fluid and spinal nerves	
Pia mater	Highly vascularized	
Spinal cord		

Note: The needle must pass through the first six layers to reach the epidural space, into which the stimulator leads are placed.

Stimulation of the back and of one or both of the lower extremities is often desired after unsuccessful lumbar surgery. Low back stimulation can most often be achieved by placing a lead at the midline between T8 and T9.[7] This is because dorsal column nerve fibers innervating L2 to L5 dermatomes are accessible at this level. Although the literature suggests the most effective lead placement for low back pain is a single midline lead, we prefer to place two leads so that they can be reprogrammed if micromigration occurs. Placing two leads, each slightly off the physiologic midline to the right and left between T8 and T10, will often allow for both low back and lower extremity stimulation. A transverse tripole arrangement is another option for capturing stimulation in the low back, although this technique currently requires placement of three parallel leads or a paddle lead. In SCS systems that allow for current steering, the leads should not be more than 4 mm apart so that current can be directed to the midline to obtain low back stimulation. When placing dual leads on either side of the midline, 2 to 3 mm of space is recommended, but this may differ for individual patients. A rule of thumb is that if the cerebrospinal fluid (CSF) layer is thin (indicated by relatively low midline perception thresholds), then the leads may be placed closer together. Conversely, a thick CSF layer would suggest a wider lead separation. When unilateral lower extremity stimulation is desired, the lead is usually placed slightly off the midline somewhere between T9 and T11. By placing one lead at the midline and a second lead 2 to 4 mm off the midline, current can be steered from medial to lateral as well as cephalad to caudal such that the posterior thigh, anterior thigh,

buttock, or calf can often be selectively targeted. Distal lower extremity stimulation, such as to a foot, is usually achievable and often requires that the lead be placed near the level of the conus between T12 and L1, usually 1 to 4 mm off the midline. If foot or pelvic stimulation cannot be achieved using antegrade lead placement or if rectal, perineal, or coccygeal stimulation is desired, the lead may have to be placed retrograde and the lumbosacral roots stimulated. Spinal nerve root stimulation will not be covered in this book. Again, lateral fluoroscopy should always be performed to document placement of the leads within the cervical or thoracic epidural space.

Loss-of-Resistance Technique

The loss-of-resistance (LOR) technique for placing the Tuohy needle in the epidural space relies on the tactical sensation from a sudden drop in resistance to syringe plunger pressure created when the needle tip is passed under positive pressure through the ligamentum flavum as it encounters the epidural space. Beginning at the skin, the Tuohy needle must pass through six distinct tissue layers before reaching the epidural space (see Table 6.1). In SCS, the epidural space is usually cannulated through use of an air-filled glass syringe with low constant pressure applied to the plunger.

Some implanters use a preservative-free saline-filled plastic syringe to achieve LOR. When using this technique, the amount of saline injected into the epidural space should be minimized as it may alter the conductance within the epidural space and result in uncomfortable motor stimulation during lead testing. Additionally, it may make the diagnosis of a wet tap less clear.

We do not recommend the "hanging drop" technique for locating the epidural space. This technique relies on the negative pressure of the epidural space to draw fluid from the hub of a needle when the tip enters the space. However, in about 12% of patients, the epidural space does not have sufficient negative pressure to achieve the desired effect.[8]

The high thoracic and cervical spine may pose special challenges that require appreciation of its special anatomic features. Gaps in the ligamenta flava have been shown to be frequent at cervical and high thoracic levels as far down as the T4 level. Between T1 and T4 the ligament failed to fuse at the midline in 10% to 20% of the cadavers examined. This becomes important when entering the epidural space at the high thoracic level because the ligamentum flavum cannot be relied on as a palpable landmark to epidural needle placement above the T4 level. The significant increase in resistance that is expected when the needle tip impinges on the ligamentum flavum may not be present and a "false" loss of resistance may be encountered all the way from the laminar edge to the epidural space. Therefore, failure to realize that the tip of the epidural needle has entered the epidural space can be disastrous. As discussed below, lateral fluoroscopy is helpful, particularly in these regions.

Mechanics of the Loss-of-Resistance Technique

The Tuohy needle is placed superficially in the skin and the LOR syringe is appropriately attached to the needle hub. The syringe is typically held with the dominant hand and gentle pressure is applied to the plunger with the thumb or index finger. The hypothenar aspect of the heel of the nondominant hand is placed on the patient's back to stabilize the insertion and to minimize trauma should the patient move during the procedure. The needle should be held with the thumb and forefinger of the nondominant hand and slowly inserted into the patient's back with short milking strokes. When the drag on the needle suddenly disappears and/or air (or fluid) leaves the syringe without resistance, the tip of the needle has likely reached the epidural space. The surgeon can aspirate for blood or CSF at that time. **Note:** This technique requires special supervised training and should not otherwise be attempted.

Fluoroscopic Guidance

Lateral fluoroscopy and a working knowledge of landmarks are critical when advancing the needle through the ligamentum flavum, especially when loss of resistance is ambiguous, as it often is in the thoracic spine. Frequent comparisons between lateral and anterior-posterior views will ensure that the needle tip is approaching the midline and is not too deep.[9] Anterior-posterior and lateral fluoroscopic images should also

be obtained to document the position of the electrodes in the epidural space.

Local Anesthesia

To reduce the risk of local anesthetic toxicity, we recommend injecting the skin as well as the planned path of the needle with 1% lidocaine with epinephrine, 1:200,000 (methylparaben-free). As much as 7 mg/kg of lidocaine mixed with epinephrine (42 mL in a 60-kg adult) can be injected subcutaneously with minimal risk of toxicity. Lidocaine is preferred over bupivacaine because of its reduced cardiotoxicity should there be an inadvertent intravascular injection.

Anesthesia

Minimal sedation should be used during the procedure. The patient needs to be alert and communicative during intraoperative stimulation testing to ensure proper positioning of the leads.[9] Implanters must always be ready to deal with complications. Airway equipment, resuscitation drugs, oxygen, and resuscitation equipment must be maintained and readily available.

Management During the Trial

Trials of SCS, usually conducted on an outpatient basis, normally last 3 to 8 days, although the range may extend from 1 day in certain cases to several weeks in others, particularly when the lead has been tunneled laterally, to minimize infection risk. Some physicians perform a trial on the table and proceed immediately to permanent implantation if the patient responds favorably. We favor a 7-day trial because it adequately assesses efficacy, predicts short-term failure, and reduces the risk of infection.[1,2]

Patients undergoing cervical trials should be fitted with a cervical collar to minimize neck movement, which could lead to migration. Some implanters also use a back brace for lumbar trials, although we have not had a problem with lumbar SCS leads migrating as long as the patient is educated with regard to bending, reaching, and proper motion. We prefer outpatient trials because they are more representative of what the patient will encounter should a permanent implant be indicated. Frequent monitoring during the trial is necessary to ensure that paresthesia coverage continues to be optimal and that the patient is comfortable with the equipment. The clinical specialist or manufacturer must be easily accessible so that simple corrections in programming can be performed promptly if needed. If the patient has difficulty contacting the clinic or specialist in a timely manner, he or she will lose confidence in the clinic or specialist's ability to provide reliable customer service and will not want to proceed to permanent implantation. Remember, if the patient is disappointed with the results of the trial, for whatever reason, it is very unlikely that he or she will ever consider neuromodulation in the future.

Assessment of Trial

A successful trial is customarily defined as one that reduces the patient's pain by 50% from its pretrial level, as measured on an 11-point visual analog scale (VAS). This number is actually quite arbitrary, without any intrinsic significance. Data in support of this number are lacking. In fact, evidence shows that patients who report higher levels of relief (70% and higher) have a greater likelihood of sustained relief with a permanent implant.[10] There is also evidence that changes in VAS scores of at least 20 on a 100-mm scale, or a 30% reduction, are significant.[11]

How can we compare a 50% reduction in ischemic pain or angina to a 50% reduction in radiculitis? It is difficult to draw any hard conclusions based on the subjectivity of the scores and the variability from patient to patient. It makes more sense to incorporate functional measures into the assessment because functional improvement will more likely translate into improvements in quality of life than isolated pain ratings. When assessing the results of a trial, we feel that evidence of functional improvement (e.g., increased ability to walk, doing household chores, and obtaining more restful sleep) carries just as much weight, if not more, than the percentage of pain relief.

REFERENCES

1. North RB. SCS trial duration [editorial]. *Neuromodulation* 2003;6:4–5.
2. Weinand ME, Madhusudan H, Davis B, et al. Acute vs. prolonged screening for spinal cord stimulation in chronic pain. *Neuromodulation* 2003;6(1):15–9.
3. DuPen SL, Peterson DG, Bogosian AC, et al. A new permanent exteriorized epidural catheter for narcotic self-administration to control cancer pain. *Cancer* 1987;59(5):986–93.
4. Kumar K, Hunter G. Spinal epidural abscess. *Neurocrit Care* 2005;2(3):245–51.
5. Barolat G. Experience with 509 plate electrodes implanted epidurally from C1 to L1. *Stereotact Funct Neurosurg* 1993;61(2):60–79.
6. Stojanovic MP, Abdi S. Spinal cord stimulation. *Pain Physician* 2002;5:156–66.
7. Feirabend HK, Choufoer H, Ploeger S, et al. Morphometry of human superficial dorsal and dorsolateral column fibres: significance to spinal cord stimulation. *Brain* 2002;125:1137–49.
8. Ramamurthy S. Thoracic epidural nerve block. In: Waldman SD, ed. *Atlas of interventional pain medicine.* New York: WB Saunders, 2003.
9. Raj PP, Lou L, Erdine S, et al. *Radiographic imaging for regional anesthesia and pain management.* Philadelphia: Churchill-Livingstone, 2003.
10. Gronblad M, Jarvinen E, Hurri H, et al. Relationship of the Pain Disability Index (PDI) and the Oswestry Disability Questionnaire (ODQ) with three dynamic physical tests in a group of patients with chronic low-back and leg pain. *Clin J Pain* 1994;10(3):197–203.
11. Farrar JT, Young JP Jr, LaMoreaux L, et al. Clinical importance of changes in chronic pain intensity measured on an 11-point numerical pain rating scale. *Pain* 2001;94:149–58.

Further Reading

Pain and Regional Anesthesia

Lirk P, Kolbitsch C, Putz G, et al. Cervical and high thoracic ligamentum flavum frequently fails to fuse in the midline. *Anesthesiology* 99(6):1387–90.
Moraca RJ, Sheldon DG, Thirby RC. The role of epidural anesthesia and analgesia in surgical practice. *Ann Surg* 2003;238:663–73.
Nagaro T, Yorozuya T, Kamei M, et al. Fluoroscopically guided epidural block in thoracic and lumbar regions. *Reg Anesth Pain Med* 2006;31(5):409–16.

Screening Trial

Erickson DL. Percutaneous trial of stimulation for patient selection for implantable stimulating devices. *J Neurosurg* 1975;34:440–4.
Hoppenstein R. Electrical stimulation of the ventral and dorsal columns of the spinal cord for relief of chronic intractable pain: preliminary report. *Surg Neurol* 1975;4(1):187–94.
Hosobuchi Y, Adams JE, Weinstein PR. Preliminary percutaneous dorsal column stimulation prior to permanent implantation. *J Neurosurg* 1972;17:242–5.
Krainick JU, Thoden U, Riechert T. Spinal cord stimulation in post-amputation pain. *Surg Neurol* 1975;4(1):167–70.
North RB, Fischell TA, Long DM. Chronic stimulation via percutaneously inserted epidural electrodes. *Neurosurgery* 1977;1(2):215–8.
North RB, Fischell TA, Long DM. Chronic dorsal column stimulation via percutaneously inserted epidural electrodes: preliminary results in 31 patients. *Appl Neurophysiol* 1977-8;40(2-4):184–91.

Appendix A

Sample Dictation—SCS Trial

After obtaining informed consent, a 22-gauge IV heplock was placed in the patient's upper extremity. The patient was given an IV prophylactic antibiotic of (**1**), infused slowly over 30 minutes prior to the procedure. The patient was taken to the fluoroscopy suite and placed in the prone position with 2 pillows under the (**2**). Cardiopulmonary monitoring was established, and the patient's vital signs were monitored throughout the procedure. The patient's (**3**) spine was prepped with Betadine and Chlorhexidine and draped in the usual sterile fashion. The patient was given (**4**) IV for sedation immediately before starting the procedure.

An AP fluoroscopic view was obtained to identify and mark the midline position of the (**5**) spinous processes. The skin was anesthetized with 1% lidocaine containing sodium bicarbonate 1 mg/10 cc. A total of approximately 10 cc was utilized prior to the introduction of the 14-gauge 4-inch Tuohy needle. The skin entry site was at approximately the level of the (**6**) vertebral body. The needle was advanced using a paramedian approach, to the (**7**) of midline at an approximately 45-degree angle. Loss of resistance to air was utilized to verify placement in the epidural space. The epidural space was entered at the (**8**) interspace. A lateral fluoroscopic view was obtained to confirm the position of the tip of the Tuohy needle in the epidural space. Aspiration was negative for heme or CSF. The patient (**9**) complain of pain or paresthesias during the needle placement. The stylette was removed from the Tuohy needle and the (**10**) spinal cord stimulating lead was advanced through the Tuohy needle under direct visualization, medially and slightly to the (**11**) side of midline. The tip of the stimulating lead was aligned with the inferior endplate of the (**12**) vertebral body and was located approximately (**13**) mm from midline. At this point, a temporary extension was connected to the end of the spinal cord stimulating lead. Stimulator testing was performed with the assistance of the SCS device representative, and the patient reported a (**14**) pattern of capture covering the (**15**) at an acceptable voltage. The final position of the zero electrode was noted to be (**16**) from its previous position. A second lead (**17**) placed. The stylette was then removed from the lead followed by the Tuohy needle. When both were removed the position was rechecked to confirm the

lead position had not changed. Stimulation was also rechecked to verify a continued good pattern of capture. Chlorhexidine impregnated disks were placed at each of the lead insertion sites. The stimulation lead was then anchored to the patient's back with benzoin, Steri-Strips, and OpSite.

Finally, the temporary connector was attached. The patient (**18**) tolerated the procedure well and was escorted back to the recovery area. There were (**19**) complications.

The SCS device representative instructed the patient on the use of the stimulator during the trial, and again explained precautions such as avoiding getting the area wet. A pamphlet detailing additional precautions was given to the patient. The patient was reminded to notify the Pain Clinic immediately if there were any complications, such as signs of infections at the needle entry site, fever or chills, or increasing back or neck pain.

Initial stimulator settings: (**20**)

The patient understood the instructions and was scheduled to return for a follow-up appointment to assess the efficacy of the trial. After meeting discharge criteria, the patient was discharged home.

RECOMMENDATIONS

a. We will plan to have the patient follow up in (**21**) days for removal of the trial lead and a detailed assessment of the efficacy of the spinal cord stimulator (SCS) trial.
b. (**22**) medications were prescribed at today's visit.
c. (**23**) additional recommendations.

TEMPLATE

1. Antibiotic given
   a. 1 gm of Kefzol, mixed in 500 cc of normal saline
   b. other

2. Location of pillows (to reduce lordosis)
   a. Chest to reduce the cervical lordosis
   b. Abdomen to reduce the lumbar lordosis

3. Location of prep
   a. Cervical and thoracic
   b. Lumbosacral
   c. Other (describe)

4. Amount and type of sedation
   a. ___mg Versed
   b. ___mg Fentanyl
   c. ___mg Versed AND ___Fentanyl
   d. ___mg (other: specify)
   e. NONE

5. Fluoro identification
   a. C4-T4
   b. T10-L2

6. Skin entry level w/ Tuohy
   a. T2
   b. L2
   c. Other

7. Paramedian
   a. right
   b. left

8. Site of epidural entry
   a. Specify level

9. Paresthesias or complaints
   a. did
   b. did not

10. Product company name
    a. Medtronic
    b. St. Jude Medical
    c. Boston Scientific

11. Lead placement
    a. right
    b. left

12. Lead tip location
    a. Specify level

13. Lead distance from midline

14. Quality of stim capture
    a. Good
    b. Fair
    c. Poor, despite multiple attempts at repositioning the lead. Therefore, the stimulator lead and Tuohy needle were completely removed.

NOTE: For #15 and #16, dictate "SKIP"

15. Upper vs. lower extremity or upper vs. low back (axial) capture
    a. Specify location of stim capture
    b. "SKIP" IF NO CAPTURE AND SCS TRIAL FAILED.

16. Final lead position
    a. Unchanged
    b. Changed (dictate specifics of change in lead position)
    c. "SKIP" IF NO CAPTURE AND SCS TRIAL FAILED.

17. Second lead
    a. was
    b. was not
Repeat 5–16 if a second lead is placed.

18. Tolerance of procedure
    a. Tolerated
    b. Did not tolerate (describe in detail)

19. Complications
    a. No apparent
    b. Yes (describe in detail)

20. Dictate initial stimulator settings obtained from the product representative.

21. Follow-up
    a. _____ days for removal of the trial lead and a detailed assessment of the efficacy of the SCS trial
    b. _____ weeks for a routine follow-up visit to discuss any alternative treatment plan(s) given the failure of the SCS trial today

22. Medications
    a. No
    b. The following (list dose, amount, and # of refills)

23. Additional recommendations
    a. Skip
    b. Describe in detail

7

Percutaneous Trial of Spinal Cord Stimulation

Introduction

This chapter outlines the technique for performing a percutaneous trial of spinal cord stimulation (SCS), after determining that the patient is an appropriate candidate. The chapter is divided into two sections. The first describes the technique for placing trial leads for stimulation of low back and leg pain, and the second describes the technique for stimulation of the upper extremities.

Anterograde Lead Placement for Stimulation of Low Back and Legs

Patient Positioning

For this procedure the patient should lie prone on a fluoroscopic table, which will allow free access of the C-arm throughout the entire thoracolumbar spine. The patient's head should be turned to the side so that the muscles of the neck and back are relaxed. The lumbar vertebral column is lordotic, with the nadir at L4–S1. One or two pillows placed under the patient's abdomen will minimize lumbar lordosis, and all pressure points should be padded. Minimizing lumbar lordosis will greatly facilitate passing the Tuohy needle into the epidural space. Arm boards should be positioned so as not to impede lateral fluoroscopic views.

Adequate time must be taken during positioning to optimize patient comfort. Patients often have other medical conditions, such as arthritis or painful joints, that can make lying prone uncomfortable. Using additional pillows, or making modifications to enhance comfort, will allow the patient to lie still and participate in the procedure without distraction. When the surgeon is forced to hurry because the patient is complaining of positional discomfort, the procedure is compromised. The surgeon should participate directly in patient positioning as it can greatly facilitate the surgery as well as patient comfort. Once the patient is prepared and draped, repositioning becomes much more difficult.

The patient's back (mid-scapula to buttocks) should be scrubbed with antiseptic and draped as described in Chapter 4. The scrub nurse or assistant should stand beside the surgeon on the patient's left side, and the draped C-arm should be on the opposite side of the table from the surgeon.

Operative Procedure

Although the procedure for inserting temporary leads is similar to that for placing epidural catheters, the instance of false loss of resistance (LOR) is greater as a result of the larger gauge and the long bevel of the Tuohy needle used in SCS. Fluoroscopic guidance helps to overcome some of these difficulties.

To achieve stimulation of the low back and legs, the distal end of the leads (electrodes) will usually be placed in the thoracic epidural space somewhere between T7 and T12, depending on the desired stimulation pattern. The leads are inserted into the epidural space at the upper lumbar or lower thoracic spine and are directed anterograde (toward the head in a cephalad direction). A shallow, paramedian oblique approach to needle insertion is employed, and the point of entry into the epidural space should ideally be at least two vertebral segments below the lowest electrode on the lead. This provides additional stability to the lead in the epidural space. Because the tip of the lead will usually be between T7 and T12, the epidural space is usually entered between the T12–L1 and L2–L3 interlaminar space. All things being equal, entering between the L2 and L3 levels is technically safest because the conus of the spinal cord is cephalad to L2–L3 in most adults.

Several methods for needle placement have been described. We recommend using specific landmarks to eliminate the guesswork when identifying the needle entry point needed to obtain the correct oblique 30- to 45-degree needle angle required to facilitate lead steering.[1–4] Described here is a reproducible technique that can be applied to most average-sized patients and can be used for placement of the 14-gauge Tuohy needle in the lumbar or thoracic spine.

1. Anteroposterior (AP) alignment: Align the fluoroscope in an AP projection such that the spinous processes are precisely midway between the pedicles on either side. If the patient is scoliotic, align the spinous process at the level of the interlaminar space being entered.

2. Align vertebral endplates: Align the vertebral endplates at the level of the desired intralaminar entry site so that they are horizontal, crisp, and linear. Pedicles are highlighted in Figure 7.1. Radiologists refer to this as an orthogonal view, which is defined as having a set of mutually perpendicular axes meeting at right angles. This approach avoids producing a parallax error (see Chapter 3).

3. Skin entry: In an average-sized adult, the skin entry will be at the medial aspect of the ipsilateral pedicle below the interlaminar space being entered (i.e., 9 o'clock or 3 o'clock position on the pedicle).

When the insertion point is selected, the tip of a pair of scissors or marker is placed over the point to provide a fluoroscopic landmark (Fig. 7.2). Adjustment of the entry point may be necessary in patients with extremes in body habitus: entry will be more cephalad in very thin patients and caudal in very obese individuals. (Figs. 7.7a & b) In our experience, abdominal obesity is not always associated with proportional girth in the back. We will generally use the pedicle as an initial landmark and adjust the insertion site if necessary.

4. 30- to 45-degree angle: Following intradermal and subcutaneous injection of local anesthetic, a small stab wound incision is made in the skin with a #11 blade, through which the Tuohy needle (with stylet in place) is advanced under AP fluoroscopic guidance at an upward shallow angle of about 45 degrees or less (Fig. 7.3). Entering the skin at the level of the medial aspect of the pedicle will usually result in the correct

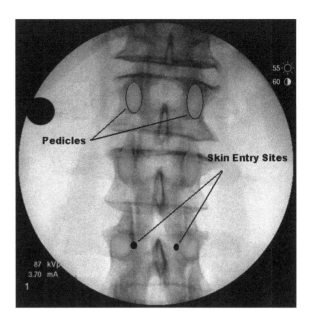

Figure 7.2 Lumbar: Selection of skin entry points.

angle of entry into the epidural space. Remember that in reality it is not the skin entry angle that is important but the laminar angle or the angle of the lead as it exits the Tuohy needle and enters the epidural space. Typically, for anterograde lead placement, entering the skin at a shallow angle will facilitate entering the epidural space at an angle that will facilitate lead steering. This line of reasoning obviously would not apply to retrograde lead placement, since the approach to the interlaminar space is reversed.

5. Contact lamina: A 14-gauge Tuohy needle with a long bevel is used and advanced with the bevel facing up (dorsal). We recommend contacting the lamina with the needle tip as a confirmatory landmark and then "walking" the needle cephalad and medial to the laminar edge. **Note:** With a true AP view and alignment of the vertebral endplates, identification of the

Figure 7.1 Lumbar: Alignment of the vertebral endplates.

Figure 7.3 Advancement of the Tuohy needle.

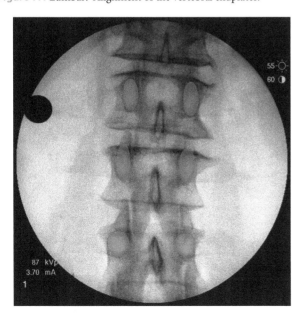

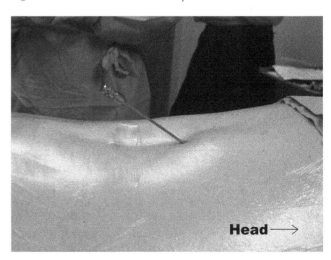

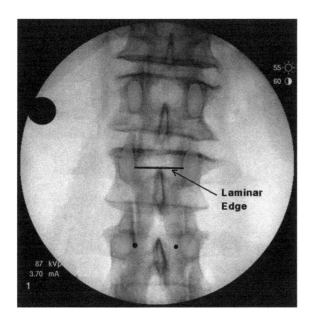

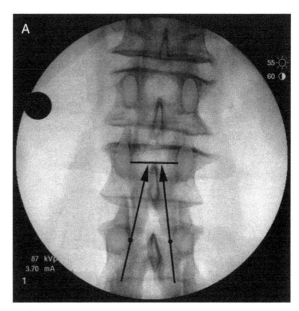

Figure 7.4 Lumbar identification of the caudal edge of the interlaminar space.

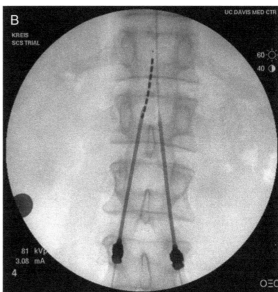

Figure 7.5a & b Bilateral Tuohy needle placement.

caudal edge of the interlaminar space is usually straightforward, especially in the lumbar spine. When the laminar edge is not clearly seen because of spondylosis, spinal osteophytes, or overlapping of the lamina in the thoracic spine, the location of the laminar edge can be inferred using the pedicle as a landmark. With a true AP projection and the vertebral endplates aligned, a horizontal line drawn between the middle of the right and left pedicles corresponds to the caudal edge of the interlaminar space (Fig. 7.4).

6. Walk off laminar edge: When the needle has contacted the laminar edge, remove the stylet and attach a LOR syringe in preparation for entering the epidural space as described above. Slightly increasing the steepness of the approach angle at the laminar edge will facilitate entry into the epidural space. Once LOR is achieved, the syringe is gently removed and the lead is slowly advanced through the needle into the epidural space under fluoroscopic guidance to verify the correct course of the lead. When placing dual leads, the second lead is introduced from the opposite side of the same spinous process (Figs. 7.5a & b) or on the same side at the next higher or lower level (Figs. 7.6a & b, and 7.7a & b). Note the difference in skin entry depending upon body habitus. (Figs. 7.7a,b).

7. Lead location: Although there is significant variability from patient to patient with regard to ideal lead positioning, certain patterns frequently recur. Most commonly, stimulation of the back and of one or both of the lower extremities is desired, especially following unsuccessful lumbar surgery. Low back stimulation can most often be achieved by placing a lead at the midline of T8. Placing two leads, each slightly off the physiologic midline to the right and left between T8 and T10, will often allow for both back and lower extremity stimulation (Fig. 7.8). In SCS systems that allow for current steering, the leads should not be more than 2 to 4 mm apart so that

current can be directed to the midline to obtain low back stimulation. Generally, dual leads, regardless of whether or not they are bilateral, are optimally separated by 2 to 4 mm. When unilateral lower extremity stimulation is desired, the leads are usually placed somewhere between T9 and T11.

By placing one lead at the midline and another 2 to 4 mm off the midline, current can be steered from cephalad to caudal as well as medial to lateral such that the posterior thigh, anterior thigh, buttock, or calf can often be selectively targeted. Lateral fluoroscopy should always be performed to document posterior placement of the leads within the epidural space (Fig. 7.9). Distal lower extremity stimulation (i.e., foot) is usually achievable and often requires that the lead be placed lower, usually 1 to 4 mm off the midline between T12 and L1. If foot stimulation cannot be achieved using anterograde lead

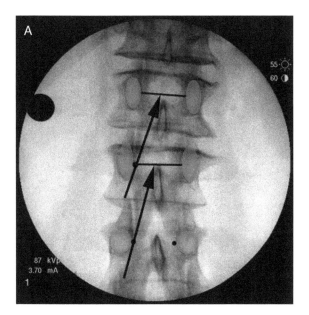

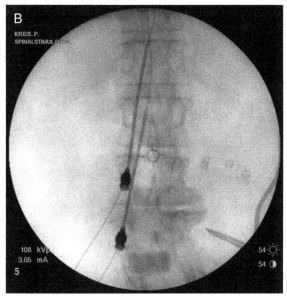

Figure 7.6a & b Unilateral Tuohy needle placement.

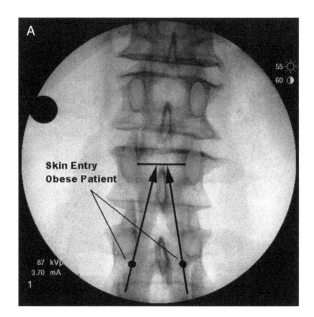

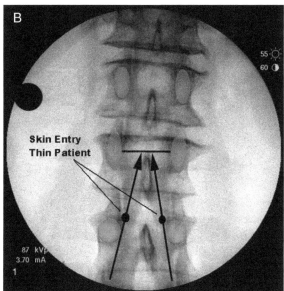

Figure 7.7a & b Lumbar entry points in (A) obese, and (B) thin individuals.

placement, the lead may have to be placed in a retrograde direction that allows for stimulation of lumbosacral roots. Spinal nerve root stimulation is not covered in this book.

Anterograde Lead Placement for Stimulation of Upper Extremities

Patient Positioning

The patient should be positioned to lie prone on a fluoroscopic table that will allow free access of the C-arm throughout the entire upper thoracic and cervical spine. The patient's head should be straight, flexed slightly forward, and supported by a gel pad under the forehead. Too much extension or

flexion will make the approach to the epidural space lead manipulation more difficult. One or two pillows under the patient's chest will promote slight cervical flexion, and all pressure points should be padded. Arm boards should be positioned so as not to get in the way of lateral fluoroscopic views. For this type of lead placement, supplemental oxygen should be administered because air circulation may be suboptimal given the head position and draping. The patient's neck (base of the skull to midback) should be scrubbed with antiseptic and draped as described in Chapter 4. The scrub nurse should stand beside the surgeon on the patient's left side, and the draped C-arm should be opposite the table from the surgeon.

The issues mentioned earlier regarding positioning and comfort of the patient apply to lead placement for any type of

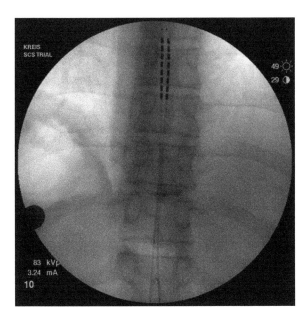

Figure 7.8 Lumbar placement of dual thoracic leads. Distal end of leads at T-8.

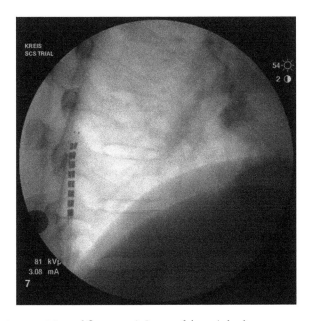

Figure 7.9 Lateral fluoroscopic image of thoracic leads.

stimulation, be it the upper or lower extremities. The importance of proper patient positioning cannot be stressed enough, as any discomfort will detract attention from the procedure itself. Positioning should be completed before patient preparation, as repositioning is much more difficult at that time.

Operative Procedure

Individuals familiar with placing thoracic epidural catheters for analgesia are well aware of the greater incidence of false LOR in the thoracic spine versus the lumbar spine. During thoracic lead placement, the instance of false LOR is even greater than normal as a result of the larger gauge and the long bevel of the Tuohy needle. Fluoroscopic guidance helps to overcome some of the difficulties associated with the greater incidence of false LOR. Because gaps in the ligamenta flava have been shown to be common at cervical and high thoracic levels and as far down as the T4 levels, LOR may not be a reliable tactile sign of entering the epidural space.

To achieve stimulation of the shoulder and/or upper extremity, the distal end of the leads (electrodes) will usually be placed in the cervical epidural space between C2 and C8, depending on the desired stimulation pattern. The leads are inserted into the epidural space in the upper thoracic spine and are directed anterograde (toward the head in a cephalad direction). As for lumbar placement, a shallow, paramedian oblique approach to needle insertion is employed and the point of entry into the epidural space should ideally be at least two vertebral segments below the lowest electrode on the lead. This provides additional stability to the lead in the epidural space. Because the tip of the lead will usually be placed between C2 and C8, the epidural space is usually entered at a level between the T1–T2 and T4–T5 interlaminar space. For example, good medial hand and arm stimulation is sometimes achieved at C7; therefore, lead entry into the epidural space should occur between T2 and T4. Some implanters routinely enter the epidural space at the T4–T5 level because there is less thoracic motion than at higher levels.

The thoracic spine normally has a kyphotic curvature with the apex at T6. The spinous processes of T1 through T4 generally project straight back, whereas those of T5 through T8 are inclined downward, potentially complicating the approach to the epidural space. The epidural space is 3 to 4 mm wide in the thoracic spine but may be less than 2 mm wide at C7. Marked scoliosis can twist the spine, increasing the technical difficulty of insertion. Unlike the lumbar spine, which contains the roots of the cauda equina below L2, the thoracic spine contains the spinal cord, and the risk of injuring the cord with a misplaced needle must be considered. Thus, the thoracic approach should be attempted only by operators who have extensive experience with LOR in the lumbar spine.

The landmarks used to eliminate the guesswork when identifying the needle entry point are identical to those used in the lumbar spine. The angle of approach to the cervical epidural space may be somewhat steeper than in the lumbar region because of the reduced interlaminar space and layering of the thoracic lamina. However, the principles for lead placement are still the same.

The description below for placing the needle in the upper thoracic epidural space is the same as for the lumbar approach. It is duplicated here for ease of reference, but the associated cervical images are different.

1. AP alignment: Align the fluoroscope in an AP projection such that the spinous process is precisely midway between the pedicles on either side. If the patient is scoliotic, align the spinous process at the level of the interlaminar space being entered.

2. Align vertebral endplates: Align the vertebral endplates at the level of the desired intralaminar entry site so that they are horizontal, crisp, and linear. In the high thoracic region, a slight cephalad tilt of the fluoroscope will usually be required to align the vertebral endplates, as opposed to the lumbar approach, which usually requires 10 to 20 degrees of caudal angulation. Radiologists refer to the aligning of the endplates as an orthogonal view, which is defined as having a set of mutually perpendicular axes, meeting at right angles. This approach avoids producing a parallax error (see Chapter 3) Pedicles are highlighted in Figure 7.10.

3. Skin entry: In an average-sized adult, the skin entry will be at the medial aspect of the ipsilateral pedicle below the interlaminar space being entered (i.e., 9 o'clock or 3 o'clock). When the insertion point is selected, the tip of a pair of scissors or other marker is placed over the point to provide a fluoroscopic landmark (Fig. 7.11). Adjustment of the entry point may be necessary in patients with extremes in body habitus: entry will be more cephalad in very thin patients and farther caudad in very obese individuals. We generally use the pedicle as an initial landmark and adjust the insertion site if necessary.

4. Shallow angle: The Tuohy needle and stylet are then advanced through a small stab wound incision made in the skin with a #11 blade under AP fluoroscopic guidance at as shallow an angle as possible depending on the skin entry site. If the angle is too steep, the transition from the needle tip to the epidural space may result in a paresthesia during insertion or cause the lead to deflect anteriorly. Entering the skin at the level of the medial aspect of the pedicle below the desired interlaminar space will usually result in the correct angle of entry into the epidural space. Remember that in reality it is not the skin entry angle that is important but the laminar angle or the angle of the lead as it exits the Tuohy needle and enters the epidural space. Typically, for anterograde lead placement,

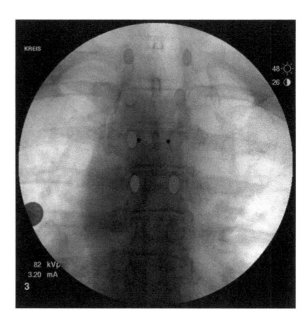

Figure 7.11 Selection of the needle insertion point.

entering the skin at a shallow angle will facilitate entering the epidural space at an angle that will facilitate lead steering.

5. Contact lamina: A 14-gauge Tuohy needle with a long bevel is used and advanced with the bevel facing up. We recommend contacting the lamina with the needle tip as a confirmatory landmark and then "walking" the needle cephalad and medial to the laminar edge. **Note:** With a true AP view and alignment of the vertebral endplates, identification of the caudal edge of the interlaminar space is usually straightforward even in the thoracic spine when the laminar edge is not clearly seen. When the laminar edge is not clearly seen because of spondylosis, osteophytes, or overlapping of the lamina in the high thoracic spine, the laminar edge can be inferred using the pedicle as a landmark. With a true AP projection and the vertebral endplates aligned, a horizontal line drawn between the middle of the right and left pedicles corresponds to the caudal edge of the interlaminar space[5] (Fig. 7.12).

6. Walk off laminar edge: When the needle has contacted the laminar edge, remove the stylet and attach a LOR syringe in preparation for entering the epidural space as described above. Slightly increasing the steepness of the approach angle at the laminar edge will facilitate entry into the epidural space. Remember that above T3 and T4, the ligament fails to fuse at the midline in 10% to 20% of individuals. When entering the epidural space at the high thoracic level, the ligamentum flavum cannot be relied on as a palpable landmark to epidural needle placement. The significant increase to resistance that is expected when the needle tip impinges on the ligamentum flavum may not be present and a false LOR may be encountered all the way from the laminar edge to the epidural space. Frequent lateral imaging is important so that needle depth can be tracked. Once LOR is achieved, the lead is slowly advanced through the needle into the epidural space using fluoroscopic guidance to verify the correct course. When placing dual leads,

Figure 7.10 Cervical anteroposterior alignment.

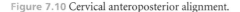

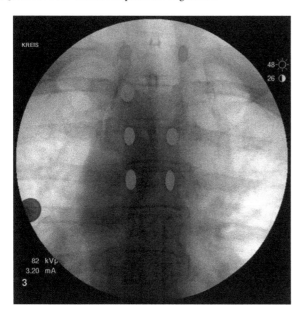

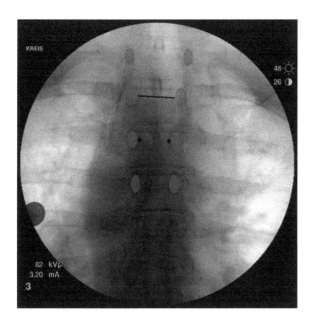

Figure 7.12 Identification of the caudal edge of the inter laminar space.

the second lead is introduced from the opposite side at the same level or on the same side at an adjacent level (Figs. 7.13a, b, & c).

7. Lead location: As in the lumbar spine, there is significant variability from patient to patient with regard to ideal lead positioning. However, certain patterns frequently recur. The most commonly desired stimulation pattern in cervical stimulation involves stimulating one or both of the upper extremities, particularly following unsuccessful cervical surgery or in patients with complex regional pain syndrome. Shoulder stimulation is often obtained with the lead placed slightly off midline between C2 and C4. Upper extremity stimulation can most often be achieved by placing the lead slightly off midline at C4 and moving it as necessary to medially stimulate the forearm or hand. Placing two leads, each slightly off the physiologic midline to the right and left between C4 and C6, will often allow for bilateral upper extremity stimulation. The image below demonstrates lead placement for stimulation in a patient with unilateral upper extremity pain (Fig. 7.14). In SCS systems that allow for current steering, the leads should not be more than 2 to 4 mm apart so that current steering between leads may occur. Lateral fluoroscopy should always be performed to document posterior placement of the leads within the epidural space (Fig. 7.15).

Lead Manipulation

Lead manipulation and steering can be challenging for the new implanter. Attending training programs that allow one to practice directing and steering leads in a cadaver can be beneficial and shorten the learning curve. We have used several different lead types and have found leads that include a steerable stylet to be the easiest to maneuver.

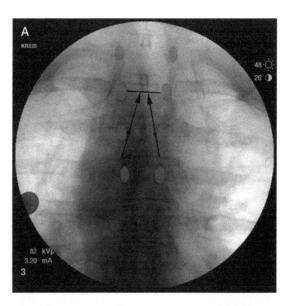

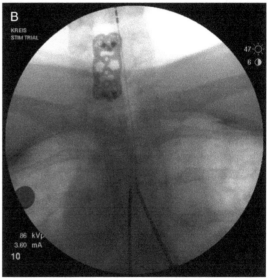

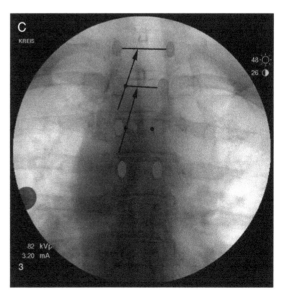

Figure 7.13a–c Cervical Tuohy needle placement.

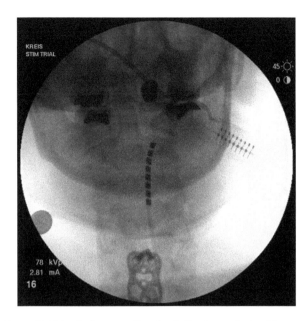

Figure 7.14 Lead placement for stimulation in a patient with unilateral upper extremity pain.

Before attempting to pass the lead, some implanters routinely use a guidewire or lead blank to establish a straight path in the epidural space for the lead to follow. Guidewires should not be used as battering rams to force through resistant or fibrotic tissue, as dural tears and other trauma can result. Whether or not a lead blank is used, it is important to try to initially establish a correct path in the epidural space because the lead will tend to follow the initial track that is created.

There are various methods of grasping and directing leads. To minimize fluoroscopy exposure and facilitate steering,

Figure 7.15 Lateral fluoroscopic image of the leads in dorsal epidural space.

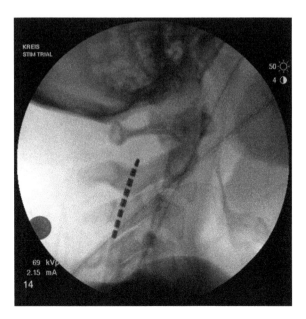

we recommend advancing the lead by grasping it with the right hand 1 cm outside the needle hub and steering the lead with the left hand by grasping the stylet steering mechanism at the distal end of the lead with the index finger and thumb. The lead adjacent to the stylet steering handle is pressed with the remaining fingers against the palm for stability (Fig. 7.16). This technique allows for a fairly natural prone hand position while maximizing the distance between the right hand and the fluoroscopy beam. In teaching many new implanters, we have found it takes a bit of practice to get the hang of holding and steering the lead.

We have learned that it is very difficult to advance the lead without the use of live fluoroscopy. When using fluoroscopy, low-dose and pulse settings should be used to minimize radiation exposure (see Chapter 3). The pulse setting can often be adjusted downward to reduce the number of images per second. We normally set the pulse mode at 4 frames per second, which is adequate for directing the lead. Fewer frames per second results in an image that is too jerky. The lead is then advanced under true AP fluoroscope positioning and frequent image acquisition or live fluoroscopy. As the lead is directed cephalad, it is important to continually correct for any curvature in the spine such that the spinous process, pedicles, and vertebral endplates remain aligned (orthogonal). Parallax error will result if the AP view is not true, which can make the lead appear to be in the midline when it is actually to the right or left. Once the lead leaves the needle it should be advanced in the midline to avoid steering into the lateral gutter or the ventral epidural space. If the lead persists in crossing the midline or exiting into the lateral recess, the lead should be completely retracted and the bevel of the needle turned in the corrective direction. If the lead repeatedly slips into the lateral recess, it should be removed completely and the needle should be withdrawn 1 or 2 cm and redirected medially or laterally using LOR. Occasionally, removing the lead stylet and enhancing the bend at the tip an additional 3 to 7 degrees or using a

Figure 7.16 Grasping the lead.

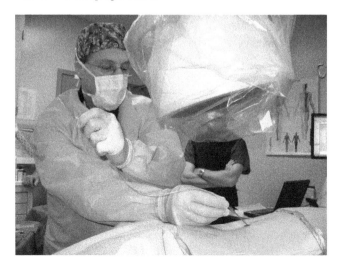

stiffer stylet (if available) can allow for greater maneuverability of the lead. If the patient experiences a paresthesia while passing the lead, it is important to stop, pull the lead back until the paresthesia passes, and confirm by lateral fluoroscopy that the catheter is in the posterior epidural space and not in the anterior epidural space. Often paresthesias are caused by lateral or anterior placement. If the lead does not pass, the surgeon should pull the lead back and attempt a new track.

Of note, one study found that lateral lead migration may be reduced by steering the lead across the midline (plica mediana dorsalis) just below the target location in the epidural space. To employ this strategy, the entry site must be contralateral and the lead must be directed up the contralateral side of the dorsal midline in the epidural space and subsequently crossed over the dorsal midline before reaching the desired target.[6]

Note: We have found that it is easiest to redirect the tip to the right or left while the lead is being advanced or withdrawn rather than trying to twist the lead or stylet when the lead is not moving forward or backward. **Important:** Never attempt to withdraw a lead against resistance, or shearing of the lead will result. If the lead cannot be withdrawn easily, remove the lead and needle completely as a unit and then reinsert the Tuohy needle as outlined above.

Intraoperative Stimulation Testing

When the lead is in position, the connector cable is attached to it and the free end is handed over the ether screen to the representative for programming. If two leads are being tested, a cable must be attached to each lead. Various combinations of anodes and cathodes, frequency, and pulse width are attempted and varied until a paresthesia covering the entire area of pain is achieved. With recent advances in technology employing joystick manipulation of current, programming can often be performed rapidly.

Stimulation testing is done with a combination of electrodes, at least one of which must be an anode (positive) and the other a cathode (negative). The initial settings for the patient with low back and leg pain usually range from 40 to 50 Hz and a pulse width of 250 to 550 microseconds. At higher pulse widths, the difference in current needed to stimulate large- and small-diameter nerves is smaller than that at low pulse widths (strength–duration curve). Patients with complex regional pain syndrome tend to prefer higher frequencies, ranging from 80 to 250 Hz. Electronically moving the cathode down the lead allows mapping of the area within reach of the electrodes. If we find a spot that covers some of the patient's pain, the pulse width may be increased to expand the coverage area. The programming units of some of the newer systems contain internal algorithms for electronically "trolling" down the lead using combinations of anodes and cathodes, making it easy to rapidly cycle through hundreds of combinations in a relatively short time.

Identifying the effective amplitude range is accomplished by gradually increasing the stimulation until the patient first reports paresthesia. This is the sensory threshold. Increasing stimulation to the point where it begins to be judged uncomfortable defines the upper limit of stimulation amplitude. The difference in voltage amplitude between these two points is the useful range for stimulation and often referred to as the comfort zone. Ideally, this difference ranges from 1.5 to 2 V.

If the patient reports that the area of paresthesia does not correspond with the distribution of pain, steering the cathode between different combinations of electrodes and varying the pulse width or amplitude is attempted first. If unsuccessful, the lead itself may need to be repositioned.

Indications that the lead is misplaced include:

- The patient feels stimulation in a nonpainful part of the extremity, suggesting that the electrode needs to be repositioned, usually caudal or cephalad
- Belt-like paresthesia around the trunk, suggesting that the electrode is too far away from the midline or too far cephalad
- Abdominal tightness, suggesting that the electrode is in the ventral epidural space
- A comfort zone less than 0.3 V or a stimulation amplitude less than 0.5 V, suggesting that the lead is in the intrathecal space or too far lateral, next to the nerve root

Anchoring the Lead Externally

After stimulation testing, the lead must be anchored. The lead is anchored externally in a temporary trial and internally in a tunneled trial, as described below. Lead migration during a trial will often result in an inadequate or a failed trial. Optimization of lead anchoring is therefore critical to the overall success of the SCS trial. This aspect of the technology continues to present challenges. In fact, the majority of complications seen in SCS involve electrode/lead failure or migration. Rosenow et al. reported in 289 patients a 32% failure rate with routine thoracic percutaneous lead placement and a gluteally placed pulse generator.[7–10]

Publications have suggested strategies for reducing the incidence of lead migration.[7–9]

Before anchoring, a fluoroscopic image documenting distal electrode location should be saved for comparison. Fluoroscopically comparing this image with subsequent ones confirms that the tip location has remained unchanged throughout anchoring. At this point, it should be confirmed that the stylets have been removed.

Most manufacturers provide several different anchor types in the lead kit. Previously available anchoring devices have suffered from unpredictable lead retention, possible lead fracture, or potential discomfort due to bulk.[10] New anchor designs are becoming available, such as a cylindrical anchor with a titanium sleeve intended to reduce lead slippage. Figure 7.17 shows some currently (as of January 2009) available anchors by several different manufacturers. Time will tell if these new designs reduce lead migration and fractures.

Use of the short-winged anchor is not recommended because it is much more difficult than the cylindrical sleeve to

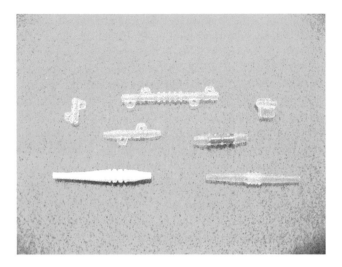

Figure 7.17 Lead anchors.

adequately secure, and in our experience it is more prone to migration. Based on computer lead stress modeling studies and consensus opinion, the following steps for anchoring the lead have been recommended:[8,9]

1. Use a sleeve-type anchor. Many have grooves or bumps on the outer surface for traction that prevent sutures from sliding.
2. Consider using silicone adhesive to attach the anchor to the lead. Injecting 0.1 cm³ of silicone adhesive between the sleeve and the lead has been effectively used in one study (Fig. 7.18).[9]

Figure 7.18 Use of silicone adhesive to anchor leads. Reprinted from North R, Kidd D, Olin J, et al. Spinal cord stimulation for axial low back pain: A prospective, controlled trial comparing dual with single percutaneous electrodes. *J Neurosurg Spine* 2005; 30(12):1412–18 © 2005 with permission from Wolters Kluwer Health/ Lippincott, Williams & Wilkins, Inc.

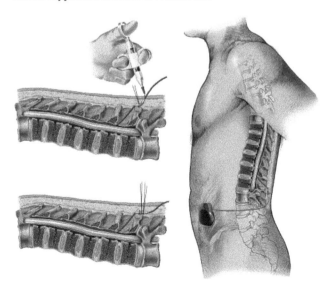

3. Attach the anchor to the skin using a figure-of-8 stitch to reduce tissue trauma with size 2-0 or 0 nonabsorbable sutures. At least one additional tie around the anchor along its length will help reduce the risk of slippage. A figure-of-8 drain tie is effective for this purpose (Fig. 7.19).
4. Consider placing Steri-Strips longitudinally between the lead and the skin along with an occlusive dressing over the exit site to further secure and protect the lead(s).
5. Repeatedly visualize the location of the tip via fluoroscopy and compare this image with the reference image to confirm that the tip has remained in position throughout anchoring. Connect the lead to the extension wire that will be attached to the external pulse generator.

An alternative anchoring technique, first mentioned by Oh et al.,[10,11] involves tying loops of silk sutures directly around the lead without the use of silicone or hard plastic anchors. Although an unknown number of implanters currently employ a variation of this lead anchoring technique, we could locate no comparative data regarding the incidence of lead migration or lead fracture associated with this method. To date, the technique appears to have been handed down primarily by word of mouth.

Due to high rates of lead migration and lead fractures associated with the use of hard plastic and soft silicone anchors, our program began to employ the technique of tying loops of suture directly around the leads by using a figure-of-8 stitch (drain tie). Lead migration was subsequently reduced markedly, especially in the cervical region, where we had previously experienced a very high longitudinal migration rate. We were not using silicone adhesive at that time, as was later described by Renard and North.[9] Although there are currently no randomly controlled trials comparing anchor techniques and migration rates, concerns about the technique of tying sutures directly around leads have focused on the potential for cutting into the insulation by overtightening the sutures being tied around the leads or other forms of lead damage.[12]

A study examined the effect of tying sutures directly around SCS leads and applying supramaximal tension (tightening the

Figure 7.19 Figure-of-8 (drain tie).

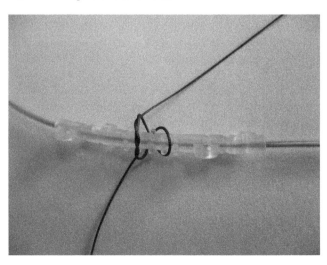

sutures to the point of breakage).[13] Two knot types and two suture types were examined. A single surgeon's knot and a single figure-of-8 knot were tied around SCS leads with 2-0 or 0 silk and tightened to the point of breaking. Examination of 28 SCS leads revealed no significant damage to the polyurethane insulation and no significant change in conductor impedance.

Although this study tested only one model of lead by one manufacturer and did not address the long-term impact of directly tying sutures around the leads or the rate of lead migration, there is now limited evidence that directly securing leads with 2-0 or 0 silk does not immediately damage the insulation surrounding the lead.[13] There is also previously published evidence that has shown that implanted silk ties in vivo gradually degrade over time. In one study, silk suture lost 30% of its tensile strength at 2 weeks, 59% at 1 month, and essentially all tensile strength at 6 months.[14] In an older study, implanted silk suture lost about 50% of its tensile strength at 1 year and all of its strength at 2 years.[15] One can therefore infer that, at 6 months to 2 years following implant, only scar tissue is holding the lead in place, and there is minimal risk that silk suture tension will further contribute to lead wear and tear. Given the limited available data as well as the unknown long-term effect of tying sutures around leads, the technique of anchoring directly to the lead must still be considered preliminary, and further study is needed to confirm and expand upon these data. Given that disclaimer, we use a variation of the previously described technique of tying loops of suture directly around the lead, which is described below.[10]

1. When anchoring the lead at the skin for a trial, first pass the suture (0 or 2-0 silk) under the lead and through the skin just at the point where the lead exits the skin. I prefer to leave the Tuohy needle in place to protect the lead as the suture needle is passed. Gently pull the suture at both ends to make sure that the suture is in secure tissue. Cut the needle from the suture. Remove the Tuohy needle and lead stylet if this has not already been done (Fig. 7.20a).

Figure 7.20a Direct anchor tie demonstration #1.

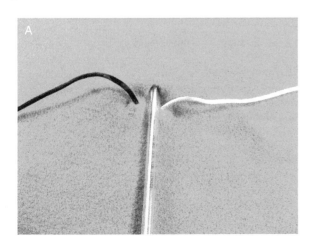

2. Tie a single surgeon's knot around the lead and tighten until it is snug around the lead. Do not overtighten, or tissue ischemia may result (Fig. 7.20b).

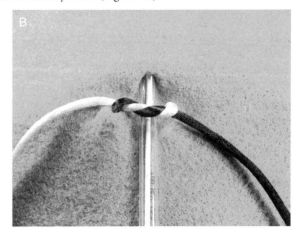

Figure 7.20b Direct anchor tie demonstration #2.

3. Tie two additional square knots (Fig. 7.20c).

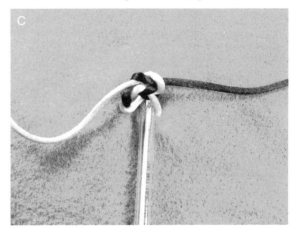

Figure 7.20c Direct anchor tie demonstration #3.

4. Wrap the two ends of the suture around the lead twice in opposite directions. Make sure that the ties are wrapped close to the original knot (Fig. 7.20d).

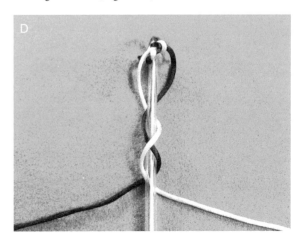

Figure 7.20d Direct anchor tie demonstration #4.

5. Tie a surgeon's knot. It is important that the surgeon's knot be very tight around the lead as this will prevent the lead from slipping. 2-0 silk and 0 silk can tolerate approximately 3 kg and 4 kg, respectively, of tension before breaking (Fig. 7.20e).[13]

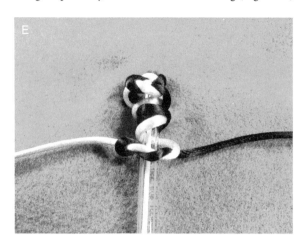

Figure 7.20e Direct anchor tie demonstration #5.

6. Tie two additional square knots (Fig. 7.20f).

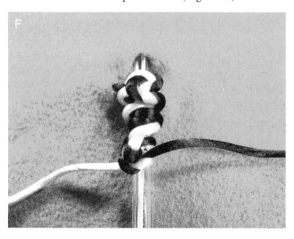

Figure 7.20f Direct anchor tie demonstration #6.

7. Repeat wrapping the two ends of the suture around the lead twice in opposite directions (Fig. 7.20g).

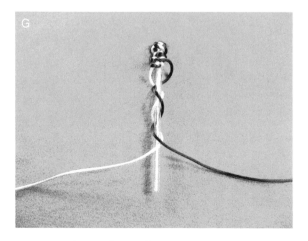

Figure 7.20g Direct anchor tie demonstration #7.

8. Tie a surgeon's knot and tie three additional square knots (Fig. 7.20h).

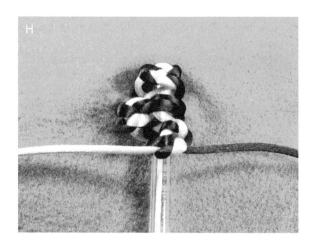

Figure 7.20h Direct anchor tie demonstration #8.

After the Procedure

After the procedure, the patient should avoid bending or flexing to reduce the risk of lead migration. The patient will be discharged after final programming and instructed to engage in only minimal activity for the first day as there may be some discomfort immediately following lead placement.

The patient should be taught how to adjust stimulation with the programmer before the procedure, and this ability should be confirmed after the procedure.

REFERENCES

1. Ramamurthy S. Cervical epidural nerve block. In Waldman SD, ed. *Atlas of interventional pain medicine.* New York: WB Saunders, 2003.
2. Raj PP, Lou L, Erdine S, et al. *Radiographic imaging for regional anesthesia and pain management.* Philadelphia: Churchill-Livingstone, 2003.
3. Andaluz N, Taha JM. Implantation of the Synergy pulse generator in the gluteal area: surgical technique. *Neuromodulation* 2002: 5(2):72–4.
4. Kumar K, Hunter G. Spinal epidural abscess. *Neurocrit Care* 2005;2(3):245–51.
5. Nagaro T, Yorozuya T, Kamei M, et al. Fluroscopically guided epidural block on the thoracic and lumbar region. *Regional Anesthesia and Pain Medicine* 2006; 31(5):409–16.
6. Mironer YW, Brown C, Satterthwaite JR, et al. A new technique of "midline anchoring" in SCS dramatically reduces lead migration. *Neuromodulation* 2004;7(1):32–7.
7. Rosenow JM, Stanton-Hicks M, Rezai AR, et al. Failure modes on spinal cord stim hardware. *J Neurosurg Spine* 2006;5:183–90.
8. Henderson JM, Schade CM, Sasaki J, et al. Prevention of mechanical failures in implanted SCS systems. *Neuromodulation* 2006; 9(3):183–91.

9. Renard VM, North RB. Prevention of percutaneous electrode migration in SCS by a modification of standard implantation technique. *J Neurosurg Spine* 2006;4:300–3.

10. Aló K. Dissatisfaction with percutaneous lead-anchoring techniques? Drain suture anchoring technique. *PRN* 2005;1(2):7.

11. Oh MY, Ortega J, Bellotte JB, et al. Peripheral nerve stimulation for the treatment of occipital neuralgia and transformed migraine using a C1–2-3 subcutaneous paddle style electrode: a technical report. *Neuromodulation* 2004;7(2):103–12.

12. Oakley J. Spinal cord stimulation and relief of pain. In Simpson B, ed. *Electrical stimulation and the relief of pain.* New York: Elsevier, 2003.

13. Kreis P, et al. Impact to spinal cord stimulator lead integrity with direct suture loop ties. Accepted for publication by Pain Medicine.

14. Stashak TS, Yturraspe D. Considerations for selection of suture materials. *Vet Surg* 1978;7(2):48–55.

15. Postlethwait RW. Long-term comparative study of non-absorbable sutures. *Ann Surg* 1970;171:892–8.

8

Tunneled Trial of Spinal Cord Stimulation

Performing a Tunneled Trial

Because incision, dissection, electrocautery, and suturing are required, the tunneled trial of spinal cord stimulation (SCS) must be performed in an operating room (OR). In a tunneled trial, a midline incision and pocket are created to anchor the lead(s) to the paraspinous fascia. The midline incision and pocket can be created before or after the leads are placed.

Once the leads are anchored to the paraspinous fascia, a temporary extension wire is connected to each lead. The extension wire is subcutaneously tunneled laterally from the midline pocket and exits the skin on the side opposite the proposed implantable pulse generator (IPG) pocket site. The tunneled extension wire prevents bacterial contamination of the midline pocket during the trial. The leads are coiled into the midline pocket for the duration of the trial. At the conclusion of the trial, the patient is brought back to the OR, where the temporary extension is removed and the midline leads are uncoiled and tunneled to the IPG pocket site.

Creating the Midline Cut-Down Incision

As noted earlier, the midline incision and pocket can be created before or after the leads are placed. The advantages and disadvantages of both options are addressed next.

Placing the Leads Prior to the Cut-Down Incision

Placing the leads prior to the cut-down incision enables ease of moving to a new interlaminar space if needed without having to extend an incision or create a new incision on the opposite side.

The main disadvantage to this option lies in the difficulty of making the incision around the placed Tuohy needles, which could cause the dissection to take a bit longer. It is recommended

that bipolar electrocautery be used when dissecting around the Tuohy needle to reduce the likelihood of conducting cauterizing electricity into the epidural space.

Operative Procedure

The leads are placed as described in Chapter 7 for a percutaneous trial. The required lead length should be determined prior to the permanent trial to establish whether an extension will be necessary at the time of permanent implantation. We recommend obtaining an actual measurement of the distance from the probable location of the distal end of the trial lead to the prospective IPG site. To traverse the distance between the midline and IPG and provide adequate strain relief, it may be necessary to use an extension. The total length of lead required should be determined before the operation is initiated. Implanters who place the IPG in the anterior abdomen often use extensions because of the increased distance to the IPG site. Ensuring that the lead is long enough will provide strain relief at the anchor and IPG sites. Strain relief is accomplished by coiling loops of lead at the anchor and IPG sites to prevent lead displacement when the patient bends, stretches, or rotates. Limited research exists regarding how much length should be added for strain relief. A computer modeling study analyzed the effect of spine flexion on the distance between an IPG implanted in the buttock and the midline anchor. In this study, spine flexion increased the distance between the IPG and anchor by 9 cm. Based on this study, it seems reasonable to recommend that at least one coil of lead or extension at least 3 cm in diameter (approximately 10 cm extra length per coil) be placed at the midline and the IPG site for strain relief.[1] This may reduce lead tension during spine flexion and possibly reduce migration. When it comes to strain relief, it is better to overestimate the length of lead that will be required.

Permanent leads can often be tunneled directly without the use of extensions when IPGs are placed in the gluteal region for lumbar SCS or in the mid-axillary region for cervical SCS.

We routinely use 70-cm leads and, if possible, tunnel directly to the IPG at the time of the permanent implant without extensions in order to reduce both the number of electrical connections and the tethering effect of an extension connector.

The leads for a permanent trial are anchored internally, as described here.

Choosing Incision Location

Depending on whether one or two leads have been placed in the epidural space, there are several options for placing the skin incision to create the midline pocket. A reference anteroposterior (AP) fluoroscopic image should be saved and the location of the lead's tip should be noted to confirm that the position remains unchanged throughout anchoring.

Withdraw the Tuohy needles approximately 2 cm while stabilizing the lead and confirm via lateral fluoroscopy that the needle tips are posterior to the epidural space. This will help to prevent inadvertent advancement of the Tuohy needle through the dura during dissection. Do not remove the needle shafts completely, as they provide lead protection during pocket dissection. Withdrawing the Tuohy needles at least 2 cm will also prevent current from being carried to the epidural space during electrocautery. Bipolar electrocautery is also recommended to avoid any possibility of conducting current to the epidural space via the Tuohy needle.

Note: We have never had a patient experience an electric shock with unipolar electrocautery as long as the Tuohy needle is pulled back sufficiently away from the epidural space prior to midline pocket creation. Adequate needle retraction ensures that electricity will not be conducted to the epidural space unless, of course, the insulation around the lead is torn or damaged, which would allow a short circuit to occur.

One-Lead Placement

If only one lead has been placed, the pocket is simply created at the skin exit site of the needle by creating a vertical incision 2 cm above and below the needle. A pocket is created by dissecting the subcutaneous tissue on either side of the needle down to (but not through) the paraspinous fascia and undermined laterally 1cm on each side of the needle (see below – Creating the Central Pocket). Once the dissection is completed, the Tuohy needle is carefully removed over the lead while the lead is stabilized with the opposite hand to prevent movement. The lead stylet is then removed before sliding the needle off the end of the lead. Fluoroscopy is used to verify unchanged lead position prior to anchoring.

Two-Lead Placement

If two leads have been placed, then the location of the exiting Tuohy needles determines the midline pocket incision location. Different scenarios are outlined here.

Two Needles at Same Vertebral Level on Opposite Sides of Midline

Option A: Placing a Single Vertical Incision Between the Two Needles (Fig. 8.1)

Following infiltration of the skin with local anesthetic, the skin is incised vertically in the midline between the two needles over the spinous processes. The incision should extend 2 cm above an imaginary line drawn between the two needles at the skin entry point and 2 cm below. A pocket is then dissected through the subcutaneous tissue and undermined laterally, thereby exposing the needle shafts within the pocket. Following dissection and control of bleeding, the needle is carefully removed while the lead is stabilized with the opposite hand to prevent movement. The lead stylets are then removed before sliding the needles off the end of the leads. The first lead is then grasped with DeBakey forceps where it exits the tissue within the pocket to stabilize the lead and prevent movement. The lead is pushed from the outside through the exit site into the pocket so that the entire lead is within the pocket. The procedure is repeated for the other lead. Fluoroscopy should be used to verify unchanged lead position.

Option B: Use a Transverse Incision, Thereby Incorporating the Needles into the Incision (Fig. 8.2)

Following infiltration of the skin with local anesthetic, the skin is incised horizontally, incorporating the two needles into

Figure 8.1 Single midline incision.

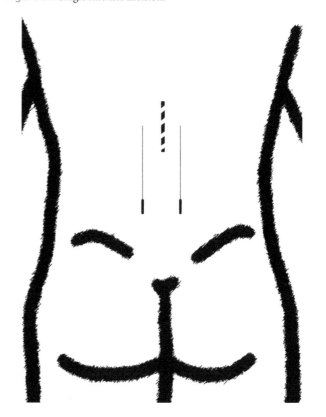

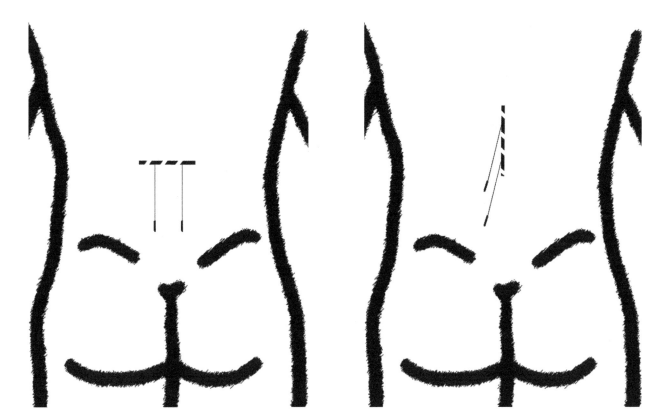

Figure 8.2 Transverse incision.

Figure 8.3 Single vertical incision.

the incision. The incision should extend 1 cm lateral to each needle. Dissecting the subcutaneous tissue between the needles on each side creates a horizontal pocket. Following dissection and control of bleeding, each needle is then carefully removed while the lead is stabilized with the opposite hand to prevent movement. The lead stylets are then removed before sliding the needles off the end of the leads. Fluoroscopy should be used to verify unchanged lead position.

Two Needles on the Same Side at Different Vertebral Levels

Following infiltration of the skin with local anesthetic, the skin is incised vertically, incorporating the two needles into one incision. The incision should extend 1 cm above and below the cephalad and caudad needles. A vertical pocket is then created by undermining and dissecting the subcutaneous tissue between the needles to the paravertebral fascia. Following dissection and control of bleeding, each needle is then carefully removed while the lead is stabilized with the opposite hand to prevent movement. The lead stylets are then removed before sliding the needles off the end of the leads. Fluoroscopy should be used to verify unchanged lead position.

When possible, we prefer placing a single vertical incision between the two needles, or placing the needles on the same side at different vertebral levels. This gives a cosmetically favorable result and places less tension on the wound than a horizontal incision (Fig. 8.3).

Placing the Cut-Down Incision Prior to Lead Placement

There are two main advantages to this option. The first is in time savings, as there is no need to dissect around the Tuohy needle. Second, making the midline incision first means that electrocautery does not need to be used again until after the Tuohy needles have been removed and the leads are securely anchored. The use of bipolar electrocautery is usually not necessary.

Although unusual, the disadvantage to this method is that one can sometimes encounter fibrosis or other obstruction, making entry into a specific interspace problematic or even impossible. If it is not possible to place leads at the planned interlaminar space, then the incision will need to be extended either cephalad or caudad or a second incision will need to be created on the opposite side of the midline. This is not a trivial matter, as an extended or unnecessary second incision increases postoperative pain and discomfort and creates a suboptimal cosmetic result. For this reason, we do not recommend a cut-down incision prior to lead placement.

Creating the Central Pocket

To create the central pocket, anesthetize the area with local anesthetic and make an incision based on one of the above options. We recommend 1% lidocaine MPF with 1/200,000 epinephrine. Incise with a #15 blade through the epidermis/dermis to the superficial subcutaneous tissue. Unipolar electrosurgery may be used if the pocket is created prior to lead placement. However, bipolar electrosurgery is recommended if there will be dissection around a placed Tuohy needle and leads. Once the incision has been made with the scalpel and the initial bleeding controlled with the electrosurgical unit, further dissection and undermining of tissue can be accomplished using electrosurgical, sharp, and/or blunt dissection.

There are advantages and disadvantages to the use of these different dissection techniques. Blunt dissection separates tissue planes without incising or cutting tissue and therefore reduces bleeding. This can also reduce the amount of fulguration required compared with sharp dissection. The liberal use of electrocautery dissection has been shown in some studies to contribute to postoperative seroma formation, but a recent prospective randomized study found no difference in the rate of seroma formation regardless of whether electrocautery or scissor dissection was used during mastectomy.[2] Forceful blunt dissection may result in unnecessary tissue trauma that increases the risk for seroma, infection, or prolonged wound healing resulting from devitalized tissue. Sharp dissection, on the other hand, results in less tissue trauma but risks greater bleeding. Because bleeding can sometimes be difficult to control when undermining skin flaps and creating pockets for the IPG, we typically combine gentle blunt instrument dissection and electrosurgical dissection in "cut" mode following the incision (see Chapter 9 — Basic Surgical Skills for the Operating Room).

Blunt dissection can be carried out with Mayo dissecting scissors, Metzenbaum scissors, or forceps such as Schnidt forceps. Mayo scissors are used for cutting and dissecting heavy fascia and sutures (Fig. 8.4).

Metzenbaum scissors are more fragile than Mayo scissors and are used for more delicate tissues. Metzenbaum scissors also have a longer handle-to-blade ratio (Fig. 8.5).

Mayo and Metzenbaum scissors can have either blunt or sharp tips. The larger size of the Mayo scissors makes them useful for undermining lateral flaps at the midline and for creating the pocket for the IPG. Forceps are also useful in blunt dissection because they have fairly blunt tips. Blunt dissection is accomplished by closing the scissors or forceps, advancing the tip into the desired subcutaneous tissue plane, and opening the scissors or forceps to spread tissue apart without actually cutting it. Care must be taken to avoid pushing the tips of the instrument through the deep fascia and into muscle or other undesired structures. Fingers can also be used to spread

Figure 8.4 Mayo scissors.

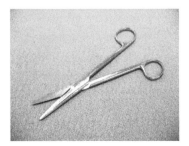

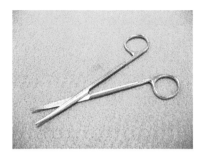

Figure 8.5 Metzenbaum scissors.

tissue to facilitate blunt dissection. Again, tissue injury caused by blunt dissection may be minimized by using a combination of blunt and sharp dissections. If it is necessary to cut tissue, small bites should be made with the tips of the scissors, or electrosurgical dissection can be used in "cut" mode. Bipolar or unipolar fulguration can be used to control bleeding. If a small arteriolar bleeder is encountered, pinch and "buzz" the bleeder with the bipolar forceps. A bleeder may also be clamped with a hemostat, which should then be "buzzed" with the unipolar electrode while in "cut" or "coag" mode to accomplish hemostasis.

Anchoring the Lead

Lead migration is the most common cause of mechanical SCS failure.[3,4] Revising a lead because of migration is difficult, expensive, and time-consuming and exposes the patient to further complications, as well as additional stress and disappointment. Optimization of lead anchoring is therefore critical to the overall success of SCS.

Prior to anchoring, save a fluoroscopic image documenting distal electrode location for comparison. Make sure that the stylets have been removed. Fluoroscopy should be used to verify unchanged lead position.[4]

The section on anchoring found in Chapter 7 is repeated here for ease of reference. As noted previously, most manufacturers provide several different anchor types in the lead kit. Previously available anchoring devices have suffered from unpredictable lead retention, possible lead fracture, or potential discomfort due to bulk.[8] New anchor designs are becoming available such as a cylindrical anchor with a titanium sleeve intended to reduce lead slippage. Figure 8.6 shows some currently (as of January 2009) available anchors by several different manufacturers. Time will tell if these new designs reduce lead migration and fractures.

We do not recommend using the short-winged (butterfly) anchor because it is much more difficult to secure than the cylindrical sleeve and, in our experience, more prone to migration. Based on computer lead stress modeling studies and consensus opinion, the following steps for anchoring the lead have been recommended.[1,5]

1. Use a sleeve-type anchor. Many have grooves or bumps on the outer surface that prevent sutures from sliding.
2. Consider using silicone adhesive to secure the anchor to the lead. Injecting 0.1 cm³ of silicone adhesive between

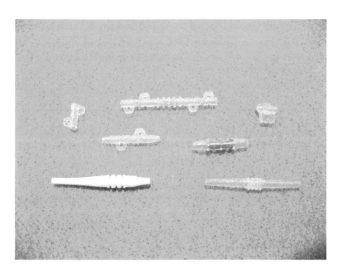

Figure 8.6 Lead anchors.

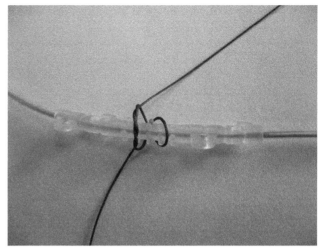

Figure 8.8 Figure-of-8 anchor tie.

the sleeve and the lead was effectively used in one study (Fig. 8.7).[5]

3. Attach the anchor to the lumbodorsal fascia using a figure-of-8 stitch to reduce tissue trauma with size 2-0 or 0 nonabsorbable sutures. At least one additional tie around the anchor along its length will help reduce the risk of slippage. A figure-of-8 drain tie is effective for this purpose (Fig. 8.8).

4. Make sure that the tip of the anchor is pushed through the fascia. This will minimize lead trauma associated with repetitive flexion and extension.

5. Place the anchor as close to the spinous process as possible to minimize lead movement caused by muscle contractions.

Figure 8.7 Use of silicone adhesive to anchor leads. Reprinted from Renard VM, North RB. Prevention of percutaneous electrode migration in SCS by a modification of standard implantation technique. *J Neurosurg Spine* 2006; 4:300–3 with permission from Wolters Kluwer Health.

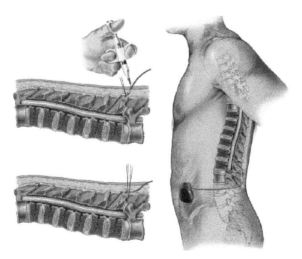

6. Upon completion of the anchoring process, fluoroscopy should again be repeated to verify that the leads have not moved.

An alternative anchoring technique, first mentioned by Oh et al., involves tying loops of silk sutures directly around the lead without the use of silicone or hard plastic anchors.[7,8]

Although an unknown number of implanters currently employ a variation of this lead-anchoring technique, we could locate no comparative data regarding the incidence of lead migration or lead fracture associated with this method. To date, the technique appears to have been handed down primarily by word of mouth. Due to high rates of lead migration and lead fractures associated with the use of hard plastic and soft silicone anchors, our program began to employ the technique of tying loops of suture directly around the leads by using a figure-of-8 stitch (drain tie).

Given the limited available data as well as the unknown long-term effect of tying sutures around leads, the technique of anchoring directly to the lead must still be considered preliminary, and further study is needed to confirm and expand upon these data.[9] Given that disclaimer, we use a variation of the previously described technique of tying loops of suture directly around the lead;

Note: We have found, as previously reported, that when using the suture loop anchor technique and creating the midline pocket, it is not necessary to dissect all the way down to lumbodorsal fascia.[8] The midline pocket should be deep enough into the subcutaneous tissue so that the leads are not palpable through the skin: depth will vary depending upon the patient's body habitus.

See Chapter 7, Figure 7.20a-h for a sequential photographic demonstration of the technique described below.

1. First the suture (0 or 2-0 silk) is passed under the lead and through the fascia at the point where the lead exits the subcutaneous tissue within the midline pocket. Make sure to pass the needle deeply enough to get a

good bite of tissue. We prefer if possible to leave the Tuohy needle in place to protect the lead as the suture needle is passed. Gently pull the suture at both ends to make sure that the suture is in secure tissue. Cut the needle from the suture. Remove the Tuohy needle and lead stylet if this has not already been done.

2. Tie a single surgeon's knot around the lead and tighten until it is snug around the lead. Do not overtighten or tissue ischemia may result.
3. Tie two additional square knots.
4. Wrap the two ends of the suture around the lead twice in opposite directions. Make sure that the ties are wrapped close to the original knot.
5. Tie a surgeon's knot. It is important that the surgeon's knot be very tight around the lead, as this will prevent the lead from slipping. 2-0 silk and 0 silk can tolerate approximately 3 kg and 4 kg, respectively, of tension before breaking.[8]
6. Tie two additional square knots.
7. Repeat wrapping the two ends of the suture around the lead twice in opposite directions.
8. Tie a surgeon's knot and tie three additional square knots.
9. Finally, we tie an additional distal tie around one (or both) leads while incorporating a loop of strain relief. (Fig. 8.9)

The same technique of tying around the leads is used as described above. This provides an added line of defense. This is demonstrated below with sequential images (Figs. 8.10a–h).

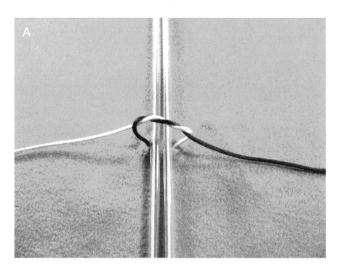

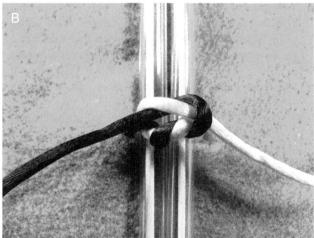

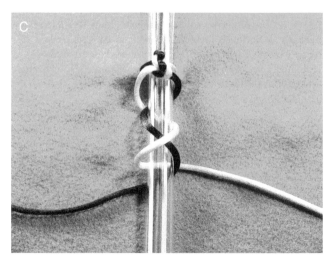

Figure 8.10a–h Tying the leads.

Figure 8.9 Midline pocket suture.

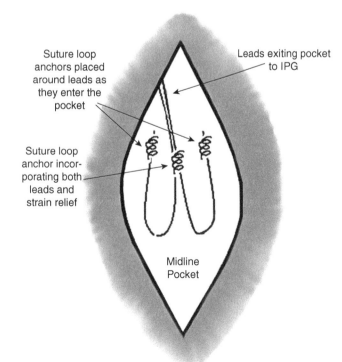

Suture loop anchors placed around leads as they enter the pocket

Leads exiting pocket to IPG

Suture loop anchor incorporating both leads and strain relief

Midline Pocket

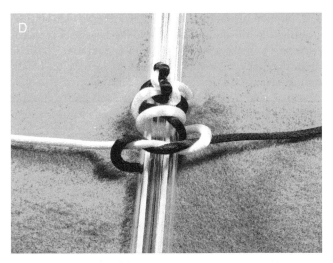

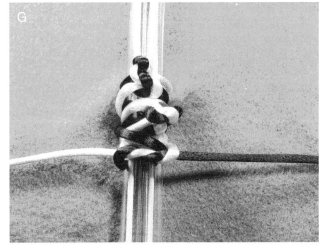

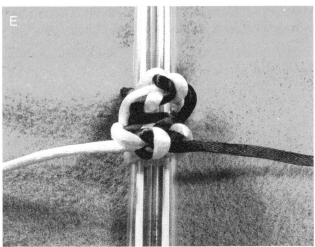

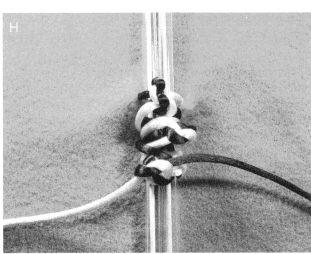

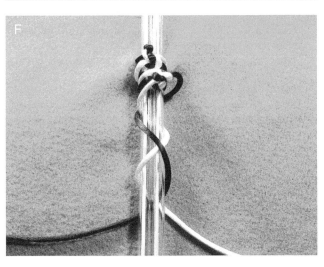

Figure 8.10a–h *Cont'd.*

Figure 8.10a–h *Cont'd.*

The Tunneling Procedure

After anchoring the lead, the extension wires must be externalized for the trial.

A tunneling tool (Fig. 8.11) is required to pass the lead subcutaneously from the midline lead anchor site to the temporary extension exit site. A tunneling tool is a sharp-tipped malleable metal probe that can be bent to conform to the shape of the patient's body. The metal probe is inserted through a clear plastic cannula sleeve (like a straw). Most tunneling tools are manufactured with the tunneling tool and plastic cannula preassembled. If not preassembled, prepare the tunneling tool by slipping the straw over the shaft and screwing the metal handle onto the metal shaft. Tunneling tools are packaged straight without any bend at the distal tip. It is helpful to place a bend ranging from 10 to 30 degrees at the distal third of the tunneling tool, depending on the curvature of the patient's anatomy. A curve allows you to direct the tip and maintain a superficial depth in the subcutaneous tissue.

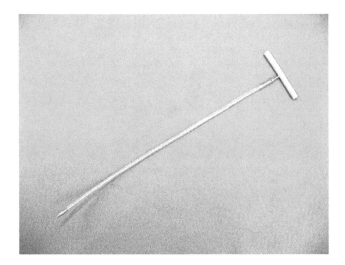

Figure 8.11 Tunneling tool.

The cannula-type tunneling tool can be advanced from the midline to the exit site or vice versa (Fig. 8.12).

If necessary, increase the patient's sedation to reduce discomfort during the tunneling procedure. Infiltrate local anesthesia along the tunneling route, from the midline incision to a point at least 15 cm lateral to the midline, on the side of the spine opposite that planned for permanent implantation of the IPG. The tunneling unit is advanced through subcutaneous tissue by applying steady force with the dominant hand. It is important to always feel the tip of the tunneling tool under the skin with the nondominant hand to gauge depth, making certain that the tip is not too deep. Steer with the bent tip to make depth and directional adjustments. The tip of the tunneling tool should be continuously palpated with the nondominant hand to be certain that it is always in the subcutaneous tissue. Vital structures can be perforated during tunneling if depth is

Figure 8.12 Tunneling. Reprinted with permission from Boston Scientific.

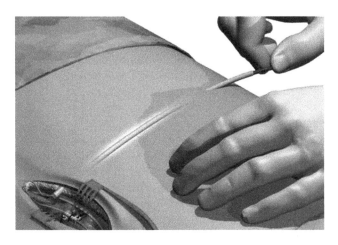

not continuously monitored. Pass the tunneling tool subcutaneously from the midline incision to the exit site. It is usually necessary to make a small skin incision with a #11 blade to allow the tunneling tool to exit the skin. Remove the handle and tunneling rod, leaving the straw in place. The midline pocket should accommodate the extension lead connector. Insert the extension wire through the straw, then pull the straw out through the exit site. After the lead has been connected to the extension wire and the connector, loop the extra length of lead in the pocket. The strain relief loops should be no smaller than 2.5 cm (1 in) in diameter to prevent kinking or damage to the leads. Generously irrigate the midline pocket with antibiotic solution. We like to irrigate with 1 L of irrigation solution per pocket. Close the subcutaneous layers as described in the wound closure section in Chapter 9. Anchor the extension at the exit site as described for the percutaneous trial. You can also place a purse-string suture at the exit site of the extension wire. Apply a secure dressing to the site.

REFERENCES

1. Henderson JM, Schade CM, Sasaki J, et al. Prevention of mechanical failures in implanted SCS systems. *Neuromodulation* 2006;9(3): 183–91.
2. Nadkarni MS, Rangole AK, Sharma RK, et al. Influence of surgical technique on axillary seroma formation: a randomized study. *ANZ J Surg* 2007;77(5):385–9.
3. Raj PP, Lou L, Erdine S, et al. *Radiographic imaging for regional anesthesia and pain management.* Philadelphia: Churchill-Livingstone, 2003.
4. Stojanovic MP, Abdi S. Spinal cord stimulation. *Pain Physician* 2002;5:156–66.
5. Renard VM, North RB. Prevention of percutaneous electrode migration in SCS by a modification of standard implantation technique. *J Neurosurg Spine* 2006;4:300–3.
6. Oakley J. Spinal cord stimulation and relief of pain. In Simpson B, ed. *Electrical stimulation and the relief of pain.* New York: Elsevier, 2003.
7. Oh MY, Ortega J, Bellotte JB, et al. Peripheral nerve stimulation for the treatment of occipital neuralgia and transformed migraine using a C1-2-3 subcutaneous paddle style electrode: a technical report. *Neuromodulation* 2004;7(2):103–12.
8. Aló K. Dissatisfaction with percutaneous lead-anchoring techniques? Drain suture anchoring technique. *PRN* 2005;1(2):7.
9. Kreis P, et al. Impact to spinal cord stimulator lead integrity with direct suture loop ties. Pain Medicine, Feb. 2009, "early view" online.

Further Reading

Screening Trial

Erickson DL. Percutaneous trial of stimulation for patient selection for implantable stimulating devices. *J Neurosurg* 1975;34: 440–4.
Hoppenstein R. Electrical stimulation of the ventral and dorsal columns of the spinal cord for relief of chronic intractable pain: preliminary report. *Surg Neurol* 1975;4(1):187–94.

Hosobuchi Y, Adams JE, Weinstein PR. Preliminary percutaneous dorsal column stimulation prior to permanent implantation. *J Neurosurg* 1972;17:242–5.

Krainick JU, Thoden U, Riechert T. Spinal cord stimulation in post-amputation pain. *Surg Neurol* 1975;4(1):167–70.

North RB, Fischell TA, Long DM. Chronic stimulation via percutaneously inserted epidural electrodes. *Neurosurgery* 1977;1(2):215–8.

North RB, Fischell TA, Long DM. Chronic dorsal column stimulation via percutaneously inserted epidural electrodes: preliminary results in 31 patients. *Appl Neurophysiol* 1977-8;40(2-4):184–91.

9

Basic Surgical Skills for the Operating Room

Introduction

Performing permanent spinal cord stimulation (SCS) implants and managing patients postoperatively require surgical skills and knowledge of wound care. Without these skills, some implanters may limit themselves to performing SCS trials while referring the permanent procedures to others. Proper surgical technique is critical to optimize outcome and ensure proper wound healing. Although technically considered minor surgery, it is nevertheless "surgery," which can be fraught with complications and devastating outcomes. Therefore, formal surgical training with an experienced implanter or surgeon is mandatory for a nonsurgically trained clinician to acquire the requisite skills to safely perform this operation. With appropriately focused training, it is possible for pain specialists without previous surgical training to safely implant SCS systems and manage their patients postoperatively.

This chapter reviews some of the basic surgical principles that are fundamental to performing permanent SCS implants safely. However, this chapter does *not* substitute for formal hands-on surgical training with one or several mentors and/or instructors. It is offered as a reference tool and an additional resource to complement hands-on training with an implanter who understands proper surgical technique and postoperative wound management. It is helpful for one to seek out a mentor known to have good surgical skills. It may be less useful to train with individuals who themselves have not had formal surgical training.

Surgical Instrumentation

The following section describes the basic surgical instruments frequently used in performing permanent SCS procedures. A basic surgical or biopsy set will normally include most if not all of the required instruments. However, the operating room manager should be consulted to determine which surgical set contains the required instruments for a particular procedure (Figs. 9.1a & b).

Figure 9.1a & b Basic biopsy set. (A) String. (B) Retractors.

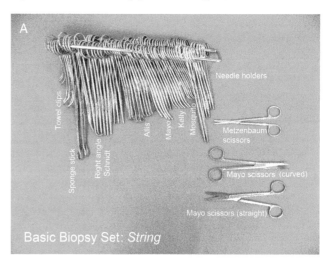

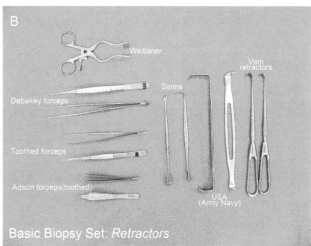

Incising Instruments

Because the length of the incision in SCS implantation tends to be small, implanters commonly use a #15 scalpel blade and a #3 handle to incise the skin (Fig. 9.2). An instrument such as a Mayo clamp is always recommended when inserting the blade onto the scalpel handle. The blade should never be attached to the handle manually because if the blade slips, it could cause a finger or hand laceration. Before making an incision, the skin should be marked to define the location and length of the planned incision. The scalpel should be held in the dominant hand like a pencil with the curved portion of the blade (belly) used to incise the skin. The tip of the blade should not be used to cut. Following adequate local anesthesia, the skin should be incised in a fluid motion through the dermal/epidermal layers just into the superficial subcutaneous tissue. Countertraction with the nondominant hand or by an assistant will aid in achieving a fluid, precise cut.

Figure 9.2a & b (A) Scalpel. (B) Blade.

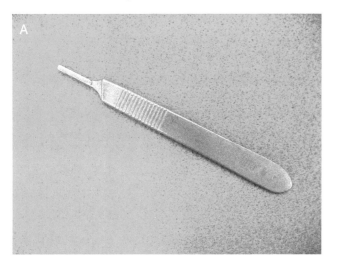

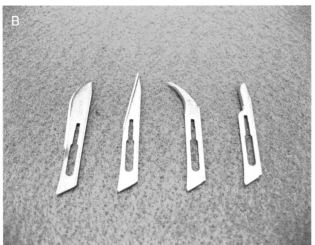

Electrosurgery

Working in conjunction with renowned neurosurgeon Harvey Cushing, W.T. Bovie developed electrosurgery in 1928. Cushing first published his use of electrosurgery in a series of 500 surgical procedures. Cushing was reputedly America's first successful neurosurgeon and developed techniques, including electrosurgery, that significantly reduced mortality, which was quite high in those days. Electrosurgery continues to be one of the most important and basic tools used by surgeons in the operating room.

Electrocautery should not be confused with the *electrosurgery*. Electrocautery is a direct-current–powered method that burns tissue using a hot wire or heating element without actually passing electric current into tissue. In electrosurgery, which uses alternating current, the patient is part of the circuit and the current actually enters and exits the patient's body. Electrosurgical equipment consists of an electrosurgical unit, and either a monopolar electrode and grounding pad, or bipolar surgical forceps that pass electric current through tissue (Fig. 9.3). When monopolar electrosurgery is used, a grounding pad is placed on the patient to complete the circuit (Fig. 9.4). Bipolar electrosurgical instruments are forceps that pass current between the two tips of the forceps. No grounding pad is required with bipolar units. Modern electrosurgical units deliver high-frequency alternating current to a monopolar or bipolar instrument.

Monopolar (Unipolar) Electrosurgery

Monopolar electrosurgery is simple and clinically effective, which explains why it is arguably the most important and fundamental tool used in the operating room. The application of monopolar electrosurgery to SCS, however, is potentially hazardous. This is because the electrons injected into the surgical site by the active monopolar electrode (see Fig. 9.4) travel

Figure 9.3 The electrosurgical unit.

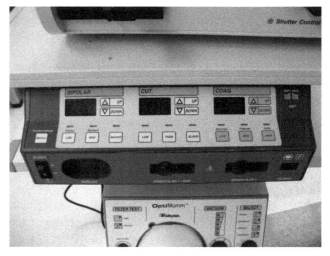

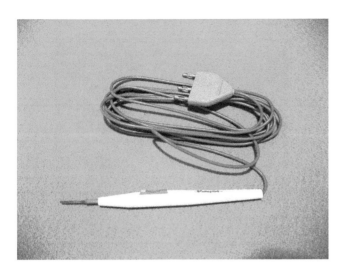

Figure 9.4 Monopolar electrode.

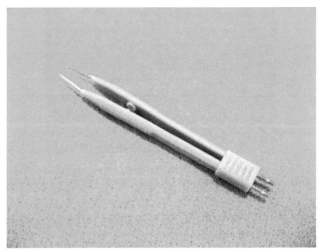

Figure 9.5 Bipolar forceps.

through the patient to a grounding pad placed elsewhere on the patient's body, thereby completing the circuit. Because current follows the path of least resistance, it may be conducted via an epidural Tuohy needle into the epidural space, resulting in nerve root or cord damage. Thus, it is recommended that a bipolar electrosurgical system be used for hemostasis during SCS implantation when a Tuohy needle is in place. If monopolar electrosurgery is used, one must be certain that a conductive object such as a Tuohy needle has been removed from the epidural space and that the insulation on the lead is intact; otherwise, current may be conducted into the epidural space. It must again be stressed that monopolar current carried into the epidural space will likely result in permanent nerve root or cord damage.

Bipolar Electrosurgery

Bipolar electrosurgery is recommended for SCS implantation because current passes between the tips of the bipolar forceps and is not directed into the patient's body, thus reducing the risk of the current arcing to a needle or SCS lead and being conducted into nerve tissue contained within the epidural space. Bipolar fulguration also limits lateral thermal tissue damage. In bipolar electrosurgery, the active and grounding electrodes are located on each of two tines of the bipolar forceps (Fig. 9.5). The active and return electrode (grounding) functions are performed at the surgery site. A short-circuit is created between the tips of the forceps. Therefore, only the tissue between the tips of the forceps is exposed to electrical current. Because the ground function is performed by one of the tines, no patient grounding pad is needed. Bipolar electrosurgery is better suited to obtaining hemostasis than monopolar because the tissue is mechanically compressed between the tines in addition to being thermally heated. It is recommended that both monopolar and bipolar electrosurgical equipment be available for every case.

Cut Versus Coagulation

Three parameters can be varied to adjust the amount of heat generated during electrosurgery: the current frequency, length of activation time, and use of continuous versus intermittent waveforms.

The "cut" mode utilizes a continuous waveform, whereas the coagulation ("coag") function makes use of an intermittent pattern. The heat generated by the cut function is focused with a high-frequency current that minimizes lateral thermal spread.

The "coag" mode delivers low-frequency/high-voltage energy, generating less focused heat and creating a larger area of thermal spread. The sparking effect typical of the coag mode results in tissue clotting and coagulum rather than cellular vaporization. The coagulation waveform produces a significantly higher voltage than the cutting current, resulting from the high impedance of air and the low frequency of the mode. The cut mode generates a higher current but a lower voltage than the coag mode. A large current reentry (grounding) pad must be securely placed on the patient's skin to prevent thermal burns at the exit site.

One might assume that the cut mode is intended only for incising or cutting tissue and the coag function is used only to coagulate bleeders. In fact, many surgeons use the coag mode to cut tissue and vice versa, depending on the desired result. The cut mode is actually well suited to thermal coagulation. Because it results in less collateral thermal injury, manufacturers of electrosurgical equipment recommend use of the cut mode whenever possible to minimize damage to surrounding tissue. By programming the electrosurgical unit, the characteristics of the cut and coag mode can also be blended to achieve the desired result (Fig. 9.6).

There is an association between overzealous use of thermal coagulation and seroma formation secondary to tissue damage (see Chapter 12). The electrosurgical equipment should primarily

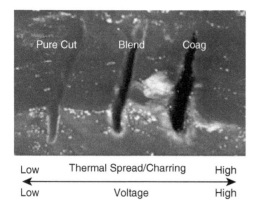

Low — Thermal Spread/Charring — High

Low — Voltage — High

Figure 9.6 Characteristics of cut and coag mode. Copyright © 2009 Covidien. All rights reserved. Reprinted with the permission of the Energy Based Devices and Surgical Devices Divisions of Covidien.

be used to coagulate bleeders and to facilitate dissection by releasing limited areas of adhesion. It is not the correct instrument to use for extensive incising and dissection of tissue planes. Sharp and/or blunt dissection will result in less tissue trauma and potentially reduce the risk of seroma, infection, or delayed wound healing.

Grounding Pad (Return Electrode)

By focusing the electrons at the active electrode, heat is produced at the surgical site. Significant current is produced at the "active" electrode that must be recovered elsewhere and disposed of safely to avoid thermal burns. What keeps thermal burns from occurring at the grounding pad (return electrode) is the reduced concentration of electrons and high conductivity of the skin/grounding pad interface. The ideal grounding pad safely disperses the current delivered to the patient during electrosurgery and conducts that current away. If the grounding pad adhesive fails or is improperly applied, electrons can be concentrated at the return electrode, resulting in thermal skin burns. To eliminate the risk of skin burns, the grounding pad should cover a large surface and should be of low impedance/high conductivity. The grounding pad should preferably be placed on well-vascularized muscle mass that is close to the operative site and away from any metallic implants that the patient may have.

Applying the grounding pad to uneven body surfaces, scar tissue, surfaces with excessive hair, and adipose or bony prominences can reduce the surface area contact between the patient and the return electrode, resulting in increased current density. An increase in current density will lead to increased temperature that can produce thermal burns (Fig. 9.7).

When using monopolar electrosurgery, the following actions are recommended:

- The electrical current should be used to cut. The active electrode tip is not a scalpel—the electrical current should be allowed to do the cutting/fulgurating without pushing the active tip into the tissue.

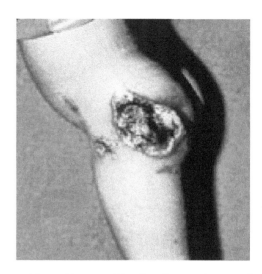

Figure 9.7 Thermal burn resulting from increased current density. Copyright © 2009 Covidien. All rights reserved. Reprinted with the permission of the Energy Based Devices and Surgical Devices Divisions of Covidien.

- The power setting should be reduced to the minimally effective level.
- Brief sporadic activation should be used and extended activation avoided.
- The unit should not be activated while close to or in direct contact with another instrument, such as a Tuohy needle placed in the epidural space.
- Bipolar electrosurgery should be considered as an alternative to unipolar because of the reduced risk of thermal damage from the bipolar technique.
- Electrosurgery, especially monopolar, may be contraindicated in patients who have implanted pacemakers or defibrillators. The patient's cardiologist, or the manufacturer of the pacemaker or device, should be contacted before surgery. Of note, modern pacemakers are often electronically shielded to protect them from damage secondary to extraneous electrical current.

Dissecting and Undermining

Sharp Versus Blunt

The following section is identical to that found in Chapter 8 but is also presented here for completeness and ease of reference.

Once the incision has been made with the scalpel and the initial bleeding controlled with electrosurgical technique, further dissection and undermining of tissue can be accomplished using electrosurgical, sharp, or blunt dissection.

There are pros and cons to the use of these different dissection techniques. Blunt dissection separates tissue planes without actually incising or cutting tissue, thereby reducing bleeding and the amount of fulguration required compared with sharp dissection. The liberal use of electrosurgical dissection has been shown in some studies to contribute to postoperative seroma. However, a recent prospective randomized study found no difference in the rate of seroma formation whether electrosurgery or scissor dissection was used during mastectomy surgery.[1] Forceful blunt dissection may result in greater tissue trauma, potentially increasing the risk of seroma, infection, or prolonged wound healing resulting from devitalized tissue. Sharp dissection results in less tissue trauma, although bleeding tends to be increased. At times, bleeding can be difficult to control when undermining skin flaps and creating pockets for the implantable pulse generator (IPG). Therefore, following the skin incision, a combination of gentle blunt instrument dissection and the use of electrosurgical dissection in the cut mode is recommended.

Blunt dissection can be carried out with curved Mayo dissecting or Metzenbaum scissors. Mayo scissors are typically used for cutting and dissecting heavy fascia and sutures (Fig. 9.8).

Metzenbaum scissors are more fragile than Mayo scissors and are used for more delicate tissues. Metzenbaum scissors also have a longer handle-to-blade ratio, which improves control and leverage during cutting (Fig. 9.9).

Mayo and Metzenbaum scissors can have either blunt or sharp tips. The larger size of the Mayo scissors makes them more useful in undermining lateral flaps at the midline and for creating pockets for the IPG. Blunt dissection is accomplished by closing the scissors, advancing the tip into the desired subcutaneous tissue plane, and then opening them to spread the tissue apart without actually cutting it. Care must be taken to avoid pushing the tips of the instrument through the deep fascia and into muscle or other undesired structures. Using the fingers to spread tissue can also facilitate blunt dissection. Again, a combination of blunt and sharp dissection may minimize tissue injury from blunt dissection. When cutting tissue, it is important that what is being cut can easily be seen and that either small bites are made with the tips of the scissors or electrosurgical dissection in cut mode is used.

Figure 9.8 Mayo scissors.

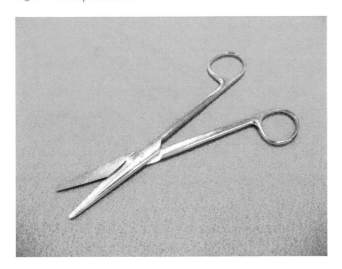

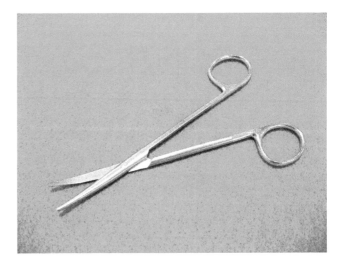

Figure 9.9 Metzenbaum scissors.

Bipolar or unipolar fulguration should be used to control bleeding. If a small arteriolar bleeder is encountered, it should be pinched and "buzzed" with the bipolar forceps or clamped with a hemostat. The hemostat should be buzzed with the unipolar electrode in coag mode to accomplish hemostasis. If fulguration does not stop the bleeder, it can be clamped off with a hemostat and a suture can be tied around the clamped tissue underneath the instrument, thereby tying off the bleeder.

Retractors

There are dozens of retractors available, and many surgeons develop a preference for a certain model. Retractors commonly used in SCS implantation are found in most minor surgical sets and usually include the Weitlaner retractor, skin hooks, the Senn retractor, and the Army–Navy retractor.

Weitlaner Retractor

The Weitlaner retractor (Fig. 9.10) is a very useful tool in SCS, especially when anchoring leads to the fascia of the midline incision. The Weitlaner is self-retaining and designed to spread and hold tissue apart using a scissor action of the handles and a locking mechanism that prevents the retractor from closing. Once the Weitlaner retractor is placed, no assistant is needed to maintain tissue exposure.

Senn Retractor and Skin Hook

The Senn retractor (Fig. 9.11a) is small and used by the surgeon or assistant to retract skin or other tissue during dissection. The skin hook (Fig. 9.11b) can be used for the same purpose. The retractor or the skin hook is used to pull the skin up during creation of a pocket or when undermining a flap.

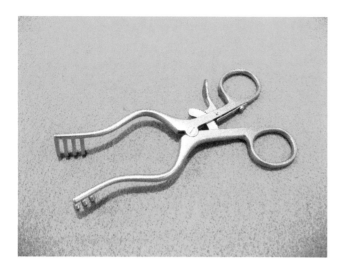

Figure 9.10 Weitlaner retractor.

Figure 9.11a & b (A) Senn retractor and (B) skin hook.

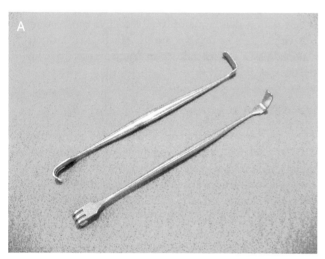

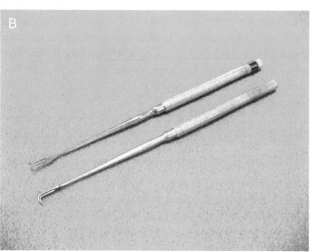

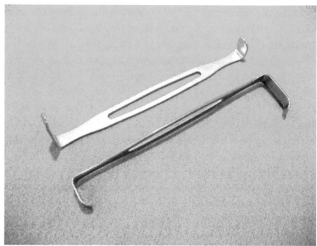

Figure 9.12 Army–Navy retractor.

Army–Navy Retractor

The Army–Navy retractor (Fig. 9.12) is larger than the Senn retractor and is helpful in SCS procedures to lift up the tissue overlying the pocket for better exposure during deeper IPG pocket dissection or examination. The Army–Navy retractor also is useful when pocket exposure is required to assess bleeding and also at the time of irrigation.

Forceps

The term *forceps* is limited to the medical arena and is derived from the Latin word *forca*, which means to snare or trap. Forceps are hand-held hinged tweezers or clamps that rely on the lever principle to grasp or hold tissue or small objects and are especially useful when numerous objects need to be clamped simultaneously. There are two main categories of forceps: nonlocking and locking.

Nonlocking forceps—such as DeBakey and Adson forceps—are commonly used during SCS procedures (Fig. 9.13).

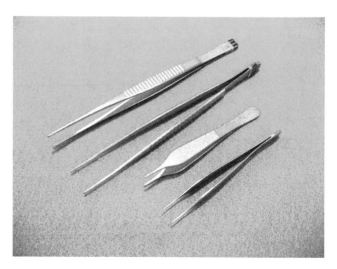

Figure 9.13 Nonlocking forceps.

DeBakey forceps are larger nontraumatic instruments normally used to pick up blood vessels or other delicate tissue and are also ideal for grasping SCS leads. They are also known as "magic forceps." Adson forceps, or "pickups," are routinely used during suturing. Toothed Adson forceps can damage leads and should not be used for that purpose.

Locking forceps, or clamps, come in various sizes such as—from smaller to larger—mosquito, Kelly, Mayo, and Schnidt (tonsil) forceps. Forceps most commonly use interlocking teeth near the handle. The locking mechanism engages as the forceps is closed, thus preventing the clamps from reopening. The teeth lock is released by a slight lateral push on the handle. Forceps are included in all minor surgical sets (Fig. 9.14).

Mosquito clamps (Fig. 9.15) are useful in stopping small arteriolar bleeds and are referred to as hemostats when used as such. A hemostat may be used to clamp a bleeder while it is subsequently touched with a monopolar electrode tip using the coag function to fulgurate.

Placing the thumb and ring fingers through the loops while using the index finger as a guide is the traditional manner of holding forceps Needle drivers are specialized clamps for holding suture needles; this is covered later in the chapter.

Tunneling

The following section is identical to that found in Chapter 8 but is presented here as well for completeness and ease of reference.

A tunneling tool (Fig. 9.16) is required to pass the lead subcutaneously from the midline lead anchor site to the temporary extension exit site. A tunneling tool is a sharp-tipped malleable metal probe that can be bent to conform to the shape of the patient's body. The metal probe is inserted through a clear plastic cannula sleeve (like a straw). Most tunneling tools are manufactured with the tunneling tool and plastic

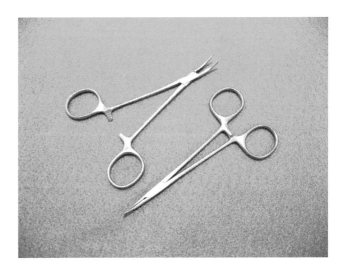

Figure 9.15 Mosquito clamps.

cannula preassembled. If not preassembled, the tunneling tool should be prepared by slipping the straw over the shaft and screwing the metal handle onto the metal shaft. Tunneling tools are packaged straight without any bend at the distal tip. It is helpful to place a bend ranging from 10 to 30 degrees at the distal third of the tunneling tool, depending on the curvature of the patient's anatomy. A curve allows the tip to be directed and a superficial depth maintained in the subcutaneous tissue. The cannula-type tunneling tool can be advanced from the midline to the IPG or vice versa. If the distance between the two pockets exceeds the length of the tunneling tool, tunneling will be accomplished in two steps (Fig. 9.17).

The patient's sedation should be increased to reduce discomfort during the tunneling procedure and local anesthesia should be infiltrated along the tunneling route. The tunneling unit should be advanced through subcutaneous tissue by applying steady force with the dominant hand. It is important that the tip of the tunneling tool be felt under the skin with the

Figure 9.14 Locking forceps.

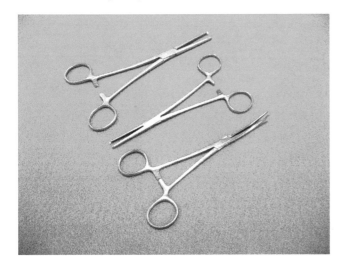

Figure 9.16 Tunneling tool.

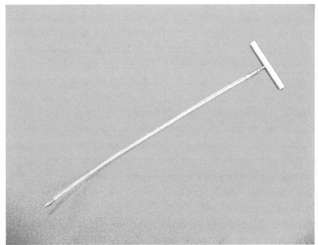

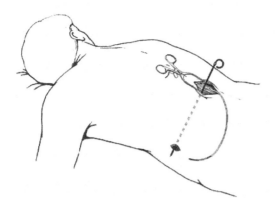

Figure 9.17 Advancement of the tunneling tool. Reprinted with permission from St. Jude Medical (Advanced Bionics Technical 10-05.ppt).

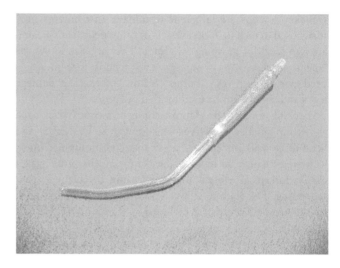

Figure 9.18 Yankauer suction.

nondominant hand to gauge depth and to ensure that the tip is not too deep. The bent tip should be directed to make depth and directional adjustments. The tip of the tunneling tool should be continuously palpated with the nondominant hand to be certain that it is always in the subcutaneous tissue. Vital structures can be perforated during tunneling if depth is not continuously monitored. The tunneling tool should be passed subcutaneously from the midline incision to the IPG site or vice versa, and then the handle and tunneling rod should be removed, leaving the straw in place.

Suction Equipment

Suction equipment (Fig. 9.18) is mandatory for aspirating blood and other secretions from the wound. A Yankauer suction tip, or a smaller tip, is usually adequate. The suction tubing can be clamped to the field by wrapping a fold of drape around the tubing and clamping with an Allis clamp, which will not perforate the drapes.

Sponges

Two types of sponges are commonly used in surgery—Ray-tec™ and laparotomy. The Ray-tec™ (Fig. 9.19a) is a small 4 × 4-inch gauze sponge that has a blue x-ray–detectable tag attached. These sponges are used to dab blood out of the field and can also be used to facilitate manual retraction. Laparotomy (lap) sponges (Fig. 9.19b) are larger and more absorbent than Ray-tec and are also detectable on x-ray. The surgeon should use only marked sponges during the operation, no matter what the size or complexity of the case. Furthermore, a marked sponge should never be cut or altered, as all of the sponges must be accounted for at the end of the case. It is the surgeon's responsibility to verify with the nursing staff that the "count is correct," which means all items have been accounted for. If the count is incorrect, the patient is kept in the operating room until an x-ray is obtained to confirm there are no retained items.

Figure 9.19a & b (A) Ray-tec™ and (B) Laparotomy sponges.

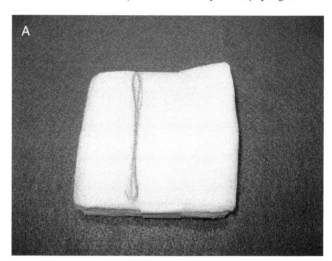

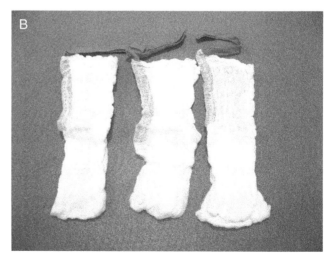

Needles and Sutures

Sutures are used to approximate wound edges and maintain a position to facilitate critical wound healing. Good suture technique and knot-tying skills are indispensable to any surgeon, including SCS implanters.

Basic Suture Instruments

Needle Holders (Drivers)

The needle holder should be large enough to hold the needle but not so large that it is cumbersome. A 5-inch Webster or Halsey needle holder is usually a good match with the size of needle normally used to close fascia and skin during SCS procedures (Fig. 9.20). Unlike conventional clamps, the jaws are only minimally jagged and touch before the handles lock.

Needle Pickups

A 4-inch (12-cm) Adson tissue forceps with 1:2 teeth (Fig. 9.21) is used to grab the needle once it has been passed by the needle driver and begins to emerge from the tissue.

Suture Scissors

Littler or similar suture scissors (Fig. 9.22) are used to cut the end of the suture after tying the knot and can also be used to facilitate suture removal because of the specialized tip.

Suture Material

Suture material is selected according to the location of the suture material (i.e., skin, subcutaneous, or deep), the healing time of the tissue, the properties of the suture material, the

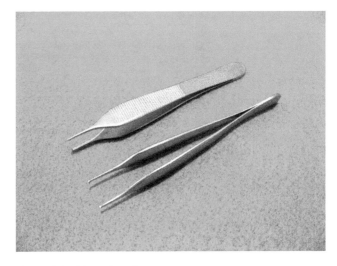

Figure 9.21 Adson tissue forceps.

type and strength of the tissue that is being sutured, the inherent wound tension and the suture tensile strength and absorption profile, and the interaction between the suture and the tissue (Fig. 9.23).

Suture Handling

The ideal suture would pass easily through tissue, easily accommodate knot-tying, and hold a knot once thrown. In reality, suture selection is often a compromise because sutures that slide easily through tissue—such as monofilament sutures—do not hold a knot as well as sutures with higher friction coefficients—such as multifilament suture.

There are many types of sutures available. Suture material is categorized as natural versus synthetic, absorbable versus nonabsorbable, monofilament versus multifilament braided, and suture size (tensile strength).

Figure 9.20 Needle holders.

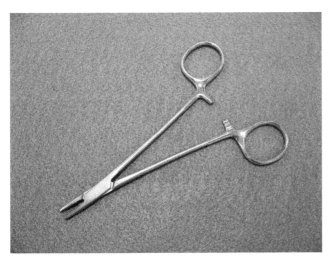

Figure 9.22 Suture scissors.

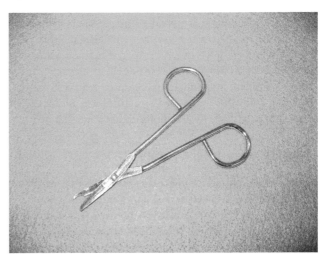

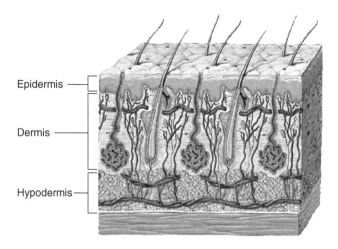

Epidermis

Dermis

Hypodermis

Figure 9.23 Skin layer. Reprinted with permission from A.D.A.M Health Solutions, Inc.

Natural Versus Synthetic Material

Natural suture is made from cotton, silk, sheep submucosa (plain gut), or beef serosa (chromic gut). Synthetic fibers include nylon, Dacron, polyester, polyethylene, polyglycolic acid, and polyglactin. Synthetic polymers do not normally produce the intense inflammatory reactions that are often observed with natural materials.

Absorbable Versus Nonabsorbable Sutures

Absorbable sutures undergo degradation within the tissues. They are designed to maintain strength for a specified period of time before undergoing hydrolysis or enzymatic breakdown and absorption. Absorbable sutures can be used to appose the deep layers and can also be used for superficial subcuticular skin closure.

Nonabsorbable sutures become encapsulated and surrounded by fibrotic tissue. When used as a skin suture, nonabsorbable monofilament sutures—such as nylon—are left in place for 7 to 10 days and then removed. Anchors and pulse generators used in SCS are secured with nonabsorbable sutures such as silk, TiCron, or Ethibond. Although silk is categorized as nonabsorbable, it is not a truly permanent material. It is gradually broken down over a prolonged period of time and after 1 year will have lost most, if not all, of its strength. Silk suture degradation is unlikely to be an issue in SCS because the leads and other implanted structures will ultimately be secured by scar tissue several months after implantation.

Monofilament Versus Multifilament Suture

The handling and performance characteristics of a suture are most influenced by whether it is mono- or multifilament.

Monofilament suture grossly appears as a single strand of suture material. However, it can be seen under magnification that all fibers run parallel and are not braided or twisted.

Monofilament suturing requires five or six knots, as compared with three or four for multifilament suturing, simply because the monofilament knots slip more easily than braided sutures. Most monofilament synthetic suture material has the bothersome characteristic of "memory"—the tendency of the suture to retain its original shape once removed from the wrapper. This makes the suture more difficult to work with than multifilament. Absorbable synthetic monofilament suture can stretch up to 30% of its original length before breaking, making it suboptimal for use in deep layers. Passing monofilament fiber minimally traumatizes tissue and resists harboring microorganisms, making it better suited for subcuticular skin closure.

Multifilament suture is made up of multiple strands twisted or braided together. It provides for better handling characteristics and easier tying than monofilament suture, with knots that are less apt to slip.

Suture Size

Suture is sized according to diameter, with 0 as the reference size. Numbers alone indicate progressively larger sutures (e.g., 1, 2, 3). Numbers followed by a 0 indicate progressively smaller sutures (e.g., 2-0, 4-0) (Fig. 9.24).

The most commonly used sutures for closure of deep layers in SCS are 2-0 or 3-0 absorbable braided sutures such as Vicryl or Polysorb. When subcuticular sutures are used to close skin, a 4-0 absorbable monofilament suture (Monocryl or Caprosyn) or a 4-0 nonabsorbable monofilament nylon suture is often used (Table 9.1).

Surgical Needles

Surgical needles must be sharp enough to pass through tissue with minimal resistance. They must also be rigid enough to resist bending, yet flexible enough to bend before breaking. Most surgical needles are eyeless or "swaged," which means that they come with the suture material already attached to the needle and do not require threading. Not only are "closed eye" needles difficult to thread, but also because of their increased width, they can cause more tissue damage than swaged needles as they are being passed through. For this reason swaged needles are preferred in almost all surgical situations.

The tissue type and the size of the wound determine the selection of needle size, radius, and shape. A needle is chosen that will allow passage to the correct depth and exit the tissue at the correct distance from the entry point. A tighter radius and more complete needle circle will allow the needle to exit closer to the entry site, which can be important when suturing

Figure 9.24 Suture size scale.

Smaller ←----------- ------------ ----------- →Larger

| 5-0 | 4-0 | 3-0 | 2-0 | 1-0 | 0 | 1 | 2 | 3 |

Human Hair   Skin Closure   Abdominal Closure

Table 9.1

Suture Types

Ethicon	Syneture
Bard Mesh	Biosyn™
Bonewax	Bonewax™
Chromic gut	Caprosyn™
Dermabond	Chromic gut™
Endomechanical	Dexon "S"™
Ethibond	Dexon II™
Ethilon	Endomechanical
Mersilene	Maxon™
Monocryl	Monosof™
Monocryl PLUS	Novafil™
Nurolon	Plain gut™
PDS II	Polysorb™
PDS II PLUS	Sofsilk™
Plain gut	Steel™
Prolene	Surgidac™
Pronova	Surgilon™
Silk	Surgipro™
Steel	TiCron™
Surgicel	Umbilical tape
Trocars	
Umbilical tape	
Vicryl	
Vicryl PLUS	
Vicryl Rapide	

All ™ marked brands are trademarks of Covidien AG or an affiliate.

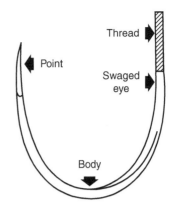

Figure 9.25 Needle diagram. Reprinted with permission from Roberts JR, Hedges JR, eds. *Clinical procedures in emergency medicine*, 3rd ed. Philadelphia: WB Saunders, 1998, with permission from Elsevier.

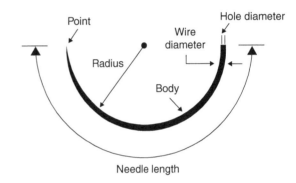

Figure 9.26 Anatomy of a needle. Reprinted with permission from Roberts JR, Hedges JR, eds. *Clinical procedures in emergency medicine*, 3rd ed. Philadelphia: WB Saunders, 1998, with permission from Elsevier.

Figure 9.27 Needle radius. Reprinted with permission from Roberts JR, Hedges JR, eds. *Clinical procedures in emergency medicine*, 3rd ed. Philadelphia:WB Saunders, 1998, with permission from Elsevier.

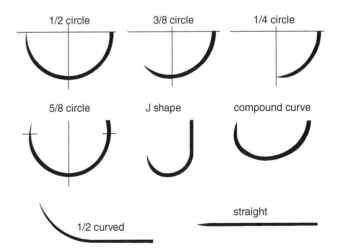

in tight spaces, such as in midline or IPG pockets during deep layer closure. Either a ⅜- or ½-inch needle is often used to close the deep fascia in SCS procedures.

Needle Anatomy

Surgical needle shapes are classified based on the following characteristics: curved or straight; needle length; taper point, cutting, or reverse cutting; radius; and amount of curve or fraction of circle (Figs. 9.25–9.27).[2]

Curved Versus Straight Needles

Curved needles are passed with a needle holder and are used for most suturing. They are more precise in "catching" the correct tissue and cause less trauma than straight needles. Straight needles are usually handheld and are often used to secure percutaneously placed lines or devices such as central or arterial lines. An instrument is not required to pass straight needles through tissue.

Taper Point, Cutting, or Reverse Cutting Needles

Taper point needles (Fig. 9.28) have a cylindrical body and a sharp tip and are often used to suture soft tissue, such as in the gastrointestinal tract, muscle, fascia, or peritoneum. The taper needle makes a small hole in the tissue through which the rest of the needle is pulled. These needles are not used for suturing skin or other tough tissue as it is extremely difficult to pass

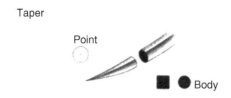

Figure 9.28 Taper point needle. Reprinted with permission from Ethicon.

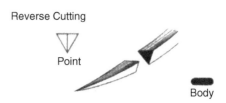

Figure 9.30 Reverse cutting needle. Reprinted with permission from Ethicon.

such a needle through these types of tissue. The advantage of taper needles is that they are less traumatic.

Conventional Cutting Needles

Cutting needles are triangular, with the sharp edge pointing inward toward the concave side of the needle (Fig. 9.29). Because the "leading" edge is sharp, care and control are required when suturing or the tissue can be lacerated. Cutting needles are routinely used to suture skin and other tough tissue. In SCS implantation, they are most commonly used in closing wounds and pockets.

Reverse Cutting Needles

Reverse cutting needles may also be used to suture tough tissue (Fig. 9.30). They pass through tough tissue just as easily as cutting needles but are more "forgiving." Because the cutting edge is on the convex side, it is more difficult to accidentally slice through tissue if the needle is inadvertently pulled up while being passed. This may, in some circumstances, decrease the possibility of sutures pulling through tissue. Reverse cutting needles are easier for beginning surgeons to use.

Skin Adhesive

Skin adhesives consist of cyanoacrylate glue that can be used in place of, or in addition to, staples or subcuticular sutures to approximate the skin edges during wound closure. They are used on the skin surface only. Skin adhesives provide good cosmetic results and can eliminate the need for removal of staples or sutures. Dermabond™ (Fig. 9.31a) and Indermil® (Fig. 9.31b) are two products currently available. Both products are simple to use, requiring only a single application; it takes approximately 30 seconds for the glue to set. Adhesives are less precise than sutures and require that the skin edges be well approximated before application. Manufacturers claim

that at the time of application the product has the strength of tissue that has healed for 7 days. The adhesive sloughs off the skin 7 to 10 days after application. We favor use of subcuticular monofilament sutures in combination with skin adhesive because the adhesive serves to seal the wound and potentially reduce infection.

Wound Closure

The ideal wound closure would result in the regeneration of tissue to its original integrity. Furthermore, the suture line would be seamless, strong, and cosmetically pleasing. Although current technology falls somewhat short of this ideal, there are many acceptable methods for closing wounds that come close to achieving these goals. Numerous acceptable techniques for suturing and knot-tying have been described. Only a few basic, straightforward techniques effective for SCS procedures are illustrated here. A more exhaustive surgical text should be consulted if learning additional suturing and knot-tying techniques is desired.

The individual layers within the midline lead and IPG pocket must be reapproximated to obliterate as much dead space as possible. Dead space can fill with blood or serous fluid, predisposing the wound to infection. By definition, there will be some dead space around the IPG, but this can be minimized by matching the pocket size to the IPG and performing a precise layered closure. The midline and pocket incisions can often be closed in two layers, especially when the incision does not extend beyond the deep fascial layer. A three-layered closure may sometimes be necessary, especially for larger wounds, and certainly is indicated when IPGs are placed beneath the fascia into the muscle layer. Placing too many sutures into a wound also increases the risk of inflammatory reaction and infection.

Holding the Needle Driver and Grasping the Needle

The needle should be grasped two thirds of the way back from the sharp end. It should be grasped 1 to 2 mm from the tip of the needle holder (Fig. 9.32).

The needle holder should be held by partially inserting the thumb and ring finger into the loops of the handle. The needle holder should be grasped in a manner that is most comfortable and affords the greatest control. The index finger can provide additional control and stability.

Figure 9.29 Conventional cutting needles. Reprinted with permission from Ethicon.

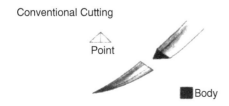

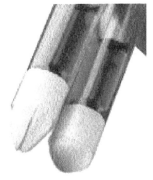

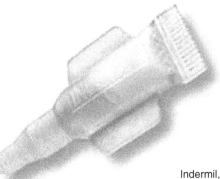

Figure 9.31a & b Skin adhesives. (A) Dermabond™ and (B) Indermil®. A: Reprinted with permission from Ethicon, Inc., a Johnson & Johnson Company; B: Copyright © 2009 Covidien. All rights reserved. Reprinted with the permission of the Energy Based Devices and Surgical Devices Divisions of Covidien.

The chisel tip applicator of Ethicon's Dermabond (left) lets the surgeon apply a broad or fine line of cyanoacrylatle glue.

Indermil, a surgical tissue adhesive from United States Surgical that requires only one application to achieve maximum strength.

As illustrated in Figure 9.33, wrist rotation is required to pass the curved needles during surgery. This motion is essential if the needle is to precisely pass through tissue at the desired point.

During suturing, small-toothed forceps such as Adson forceps (Fig. 9.34) are used to grasp and evert the skin edges. Crushing the skin edge may be avoided by using toothed forceps, which offer a secure grasp requiring minimal pressure. The forceps are held like a pen using the first two fingers and thumb in a precise pincer-type motion.

Interrupted Sutures for the Deep Layer

The first layer may be closed by using simple, deeply buried interrupted sutures approximately 1 cm apart (Fig. 9.35).

The sutures should be close enough together so that a finger may not be inserted between them. A 3-0 Polysorb or Vicryl multifilament is recommended for deep interrupted sutures. Some implanters use a continuous deep suture as their first

layer. This method, however, poses the risk of wound dehiscence if the suture breaks anywhere along its length. The needle enters the subcutaneous tissue from deep within the wound and exits at a 90-degree angle to the skin edge at the dermal/epidermal junction. The initial pass is from deep to superficial or "bottoms up." The second pass (Fig. 9.35a) is

Figure 9.33a & b Wrist rotation when passing a needle.

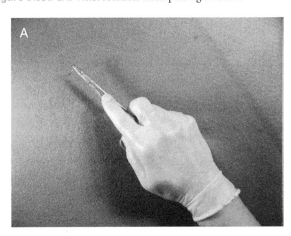

Figure 9.32 Grasping needle with driver.

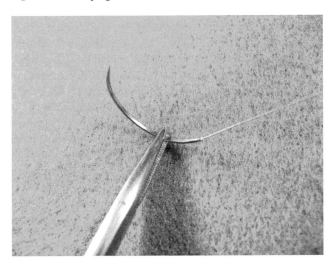

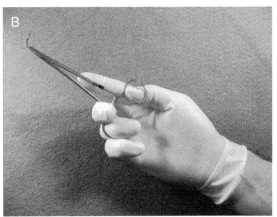

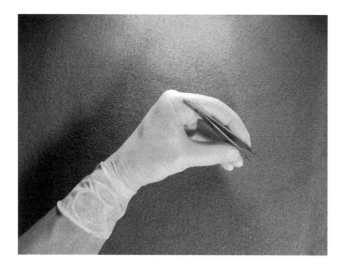

Figure 9.34 Proper holding technique with Adson forceps.

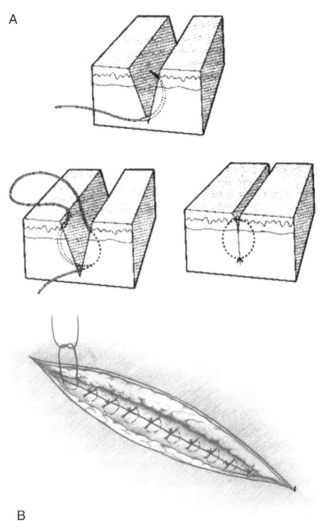

Figure 9.35a, b (A) Interrupted sutures. Reprinted with permission from the University of Buffalo, School of Medicine and Biomedical Sciences. (B) Deep interrupted suture.

made by entering at the dermal/epidermal junction—again at a 90-degree angle—to evert the skin edge, immediately opposite the exit site of the first pass. The needle then exits deep within the wound across from the first-pass entry. This will result in a buried knot. A surgeon's knot is tied and the two suture ends are pulled along the length of the incision to draw both sides of the wound together. It is important that the sutures not be pulled too tightly or tissue ischemia may result. The wound edges should be approximated, not strangulated. Three additional square knots are put in place, resulting in a knot buried at the bottom of the wound (Fig. 9.35b). The suture ends are then cut 2 to 3 mm away from the knot.

Continuous (Running) Subcuticular Skin Closure

A running or continuous subcuticular (SQ) stitch brings the skin edges together, creating good cosmetic results. The sole use of either staples or skin adhesive is preferred by many implanters, and this is certainly an acceptable closure method. A running SQ is more tedious and time-consuming but the cosmetic result justifies the additional time required. Either an absorbable or nonabsorbable suture may be used. Nonabsorbable nylon monofilament used for subcuticular closure should be removed at day 7. Nonabsorbable nylon is quite inert and does not result in much tissue reaction, which can potentially improve the cosmetic result. For this reason, plastic surgeons often use this type of closure. Nylon monofilament (4-0 or 5-0) used in conjunction with skin adhesive provides additional strength, and the adhesive also acts as a barrier to bacteria. Some SCS implanters prefer an absorbable monofilament suture such as Monocryl, Biosyn, or Caprosyn because the cosmetic result is acceptable, given the location of most SCS implanted systems. We use a 4-0 Biosyn or Monocryl on a cutting needle to close the skin, which obviates the need to remove the suture at a subsequent visit.

For a right-handed surgeon, the subcuticular suture is passed from right to left. To begin, the needle enters the dermis 5 mm to the left of the right wound corner and exits at the apex. An instrument tie is performed, comprising a surgeon's knot and five square knots; the short end of the suture is then cut close to the knot. Small bites are then taken in the dermis with the needle traveling horizontally toward the left approximately 1 to 2 mm below the skin surface. As the needle zigzags back and forth across the wound, each successive bite should enter the dermis 1 to 2 mm behind the exit point on the opposite side of the wound (Fig. 9.36a&b). This will help to prevent "dog ears" or redundant folds of tissue from forming. Small bites allow for better control and help avoid exiting through the skin. The stitches must not be interlocked. This pattern should be continued until the left wound apex is reached. It is important that the suture not be pulled tightly on the last throw; rather, a loop should be left and a surgeon's knot followed by four square knots should be tied. The loop should be cut but not the suture attached to the needle. Instead, the

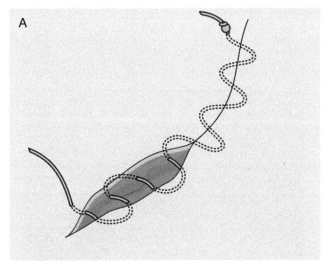

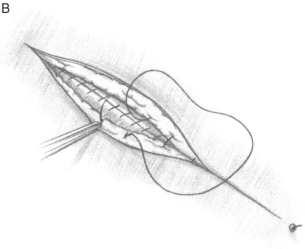

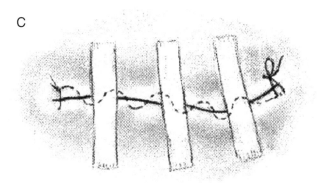

Figure 9.36a, b, & c (A) Suturing technique and (B) Running subcuticular (C) burying the suture end. Courtesy of Olek Remesz, Wikimedia. Accessed at http://commons.wikimedia.org/wiki/File:Subcuticular_suture.svg

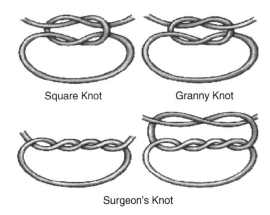

Figure 9.37 Knot types. Dorland's Medical Dictionary for Health Consumers. © 2007 by Saunders, an imprint of Elsevier, Inc. All rights reserved.

Avoid Tissue Trauma

Care should be taken to reapproximate the skin edges properly at each layer when suturing and closing wounds to minimize tissue trauma. Skin and deeper tissue that have been mishandled, crushed, or traumatized will result in more scarring and increased infection risk. Adequate time must be spent to achieve hemostasis. The use of the "cut" mode to selectively cauterize bleeders will help minimize collateral tissue trauma. Toothed forceps or skin hooks should be used when manipulating or retracting skin to avoid pulling the skin surface. The purpose of deep interrupted sutures is to relieve any tension on the skin so that wound healing is not delayed or complicated by dehiscence or infection. Tissue that has been strangulated by tightly applied deep interrupted sutures can become ischemic and necrotic, with resultant scarring, infection, or dehiscence. Thus, applying too much tension to deep interrupted sutures should be avoided. The wound edges should be drawn together snugly but not so tightly that poor wound healing occurs.

Surgeon's Knot and Square Knot

A square knot consists of two "throws," as shown in Figure 9.37. The first throw should be snug but not to the point of strangling tissue, which can result in necrosis. Subsequent throws should result in square knots that are tight but do not pull the suture to the point that it breaks. To minimize slipping, the first throw should be a surgeon's knot and the second throw should result in a square knot. The two ends should be pulled along the length of the incision until it is snug and the wound edges are opposed but not overly tight. Four square knots should be thrown with each deep interrupted suture. Five or six knots should be thrown when synthetic monofilament sutures are used. It is generally agreed that square knots provide optimal knot security. Granny knots have the potential to slip and thus should be avoided unless the intention is to create such a slip knot.

needle should be passed back through the left apex of the incision, with the exit point 1 cm beyond the apex of the incision. The suture should be pulled tightly and cut next to the skin, taking care not to cut the skin. The suture end will then retract back into the skin—this is called burying the suture end (Fig. 9.36c).

Two-Handed Surgical Tie

Two-handed knot-tying is a simple technique that can be learned relatively easily and produces a good square knot. The one-handed tie technique is not covered in this book but is available for review in other sources.

Two-Handed Square Knot

1. The white strand is held in the right hand. The thumb of the left hand forms a loop by pushing the black strand to the right (Fig. 9.38a).

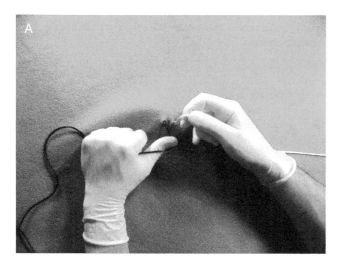

Figure 9.38a Knot tying demonstration #1.

2. The right hand brings the white strand toward the implanter and across the left-hand black strand, forming a cross over the left thumb. The left thumb protrudes through the loop that is created. The left index finger pinches the thumb so that the loop can slide onto the index finger (Fig. 9.38b).

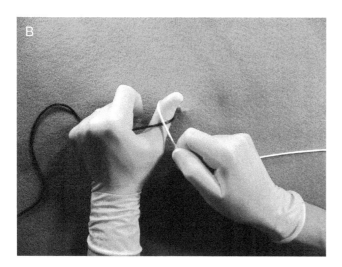

Figure 9.38b Knot tying demonstration #2.

3. The left hand supinates so that the left index finger rotates down into the created loop (Fig. 9.38c).

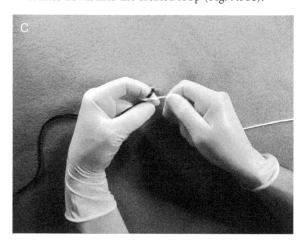

Figure 9.38c Knot tying demonstration #3.

4. The white strand is pinched between the thumb and forefinger to deliver the white strand through the loop (Fig. 9.38d).

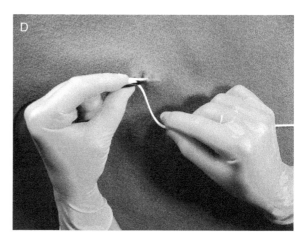

Figure 9.38d Knot tying demonstration #4.

5. The left hand pronates so that the thumb pushes back up through the loop, bringing the white strand up with it (Fig. 9.38e).

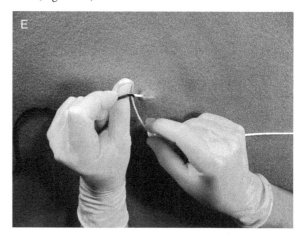

Figure 9.38e Knot tying demonstration #5.

6. The white strand appears through the loop and is grabbed with the right hand (Fig. 9.38f).

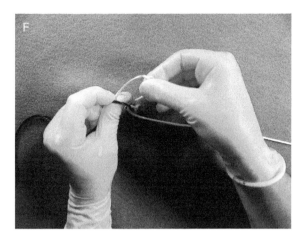

Figure 9.38f Knot tying demonstration #6.

7. The black end of the strand is tightened by pushing the knot away with the left hand and pulling the white strand with the right hand (Fig. 9.38g).

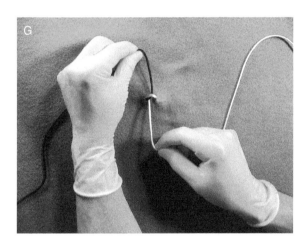

Figure 9.38g Knot tying demonstration #7.

8. The knot is pulled in opposite directions to tighten, thus completing the first knot (Fig. 9.38h).

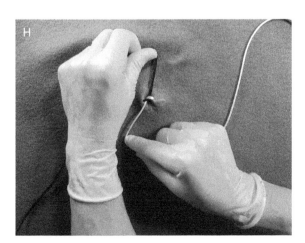

Figure 9.38h Knot tying demonstration #8.

9. A loop is formed with the left index finger by slipping it under the black strand and pushing it toward the right hand (Fig. 9.38i).

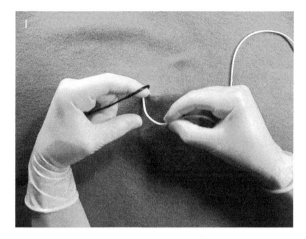

Figure 9.38i Knot tying demonstration #9.

10. The white strand is brought to the left and under the black strand to form another cross over the left thumb (Fig. 9.38j).

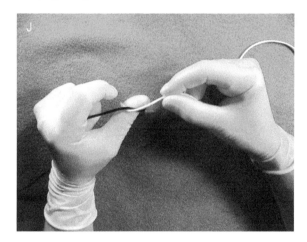

Figure 9.38j Knot tying demonstration #10.

11. The left thumb and forefinger are pinched and the left wrist is pronated up into the loop (Fig. 9.38k).

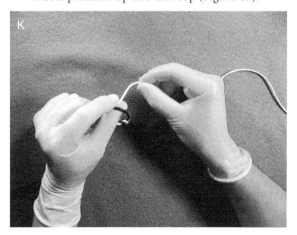

Figure 9.38k Knot tying demonstration #11.

12. The loop is slipped down on the left thumb and pinched between the left thumb and forefinger (Fig. 9.38l).

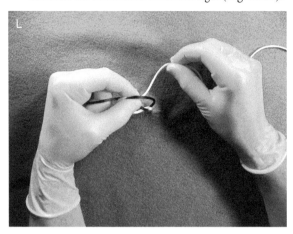

Figure 9.38l Knot tying demonstration #12.

13. The white strand is released with the right hand, and the left hand is supinated to push the white strand through the loop (Fig. 9.38m).

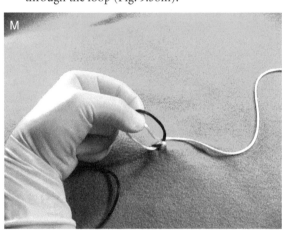

Figure 9.38m Knot tying demonstration #13.

14. The implanter should grab the white strand with the right hand while pulling the black strand toward him or her (Fig. 9.38n).

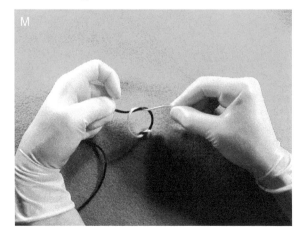

Figure 9.38n Knot tying demonstration #14.

15. The square knot should be tightened with equal tension (Fig. 9.38o).

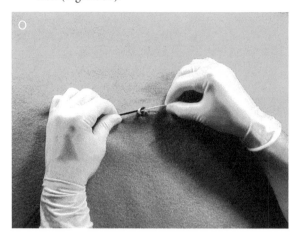

Figure 9.38o Knot tying demonstration #15.

16. A third knot should be thrown identical to the first knot to secure the square knot (Fig. 9.38p).

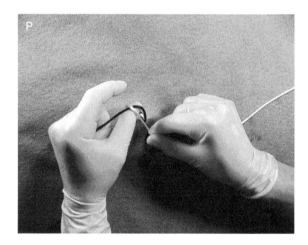

Figure 9.38p Knot tying demonstration #16.

17. After creating the loop as in the first throw, the left hand supinates so that the left index finger rotates down into the created loop (Fig. 9.38q).

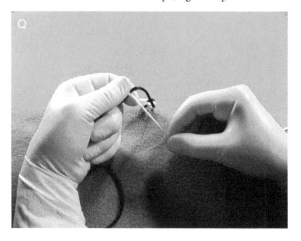

Figure 9.38q Knot tying demonstration #17.

18. The left hand then pronates to bring the white strand up through the loop (Fig. 9.38r).

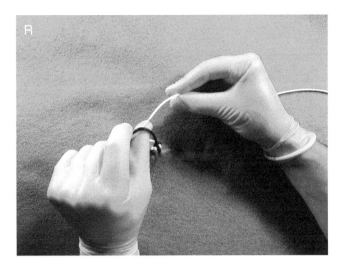

Figure 9.38r Knot tying demonstration #18.

19. The white strand should be grabbed and pulled toward the implanter with the right hand while he or she pushes the black strand away with the left hand to tighten the final knot (Fig. 9.38s).

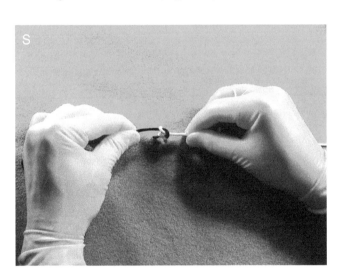

Figure 9.38s Knot tying demonstration #19.

Instrument Tie

The instrument tie is another useful alternative to the two-handed tie. It is demonstrated below.

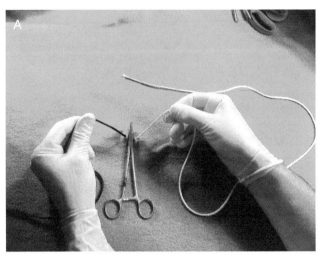

Figure 9.39a Instrument tying demonstration #1.

1. The needle holder is placed in the center of the V at the junction of the black and white strand (Fig. 9.39a).

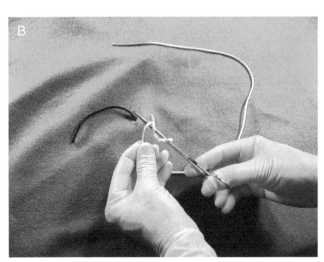

Figure 9.39b Instrument tying demonstration #2.

2. The long white strand is grabbed with the left thumb and forefinger and looped over the needle holder twice to create a surgeon's throw (Fig. 9.39b).

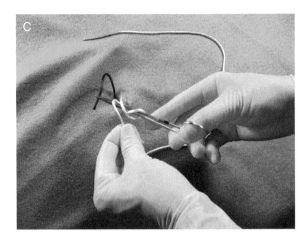

Figure 9.39c Instrument tying demonstration #3.

3. The short black strand is grabbed with the needle holder (Fig. 9.39c).

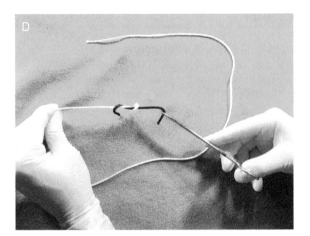

Figure 9.39d Instrument tying demonstration #4.

4. The long white strand is pulled away from the implanter and the short black strand toward him or her to complete the first throw (Fig. 9.39d).

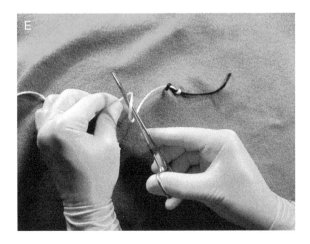

Figure 9.39e Instrument tying demonstration #5.

5. The needle holder is placed back into the center of the V again created by the white and black strands. The long white strand is pulled toward the implanter with his or her left hand, forming a loop around the needle holder (Fig. 9.39e).

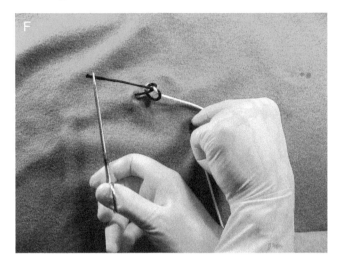

Figure 9.39f Instrument tying demonstration #6.

6. The short black strand is grabbed with the needle holder and pulled through the white loop away from the implanter (Fig. 9.39f).

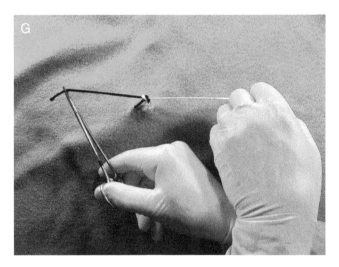

Figure 9.39g Instrument tying demonstration #7.

7. The square knot is completed when the implanter pulls the short black end away from himself or herself with the needle holder while simultaneously pulling the long white strand toward himself or herself with the left hand (Fig. 9.39g).

REFERENCES

1. Nadkarni MS, Rangole AK, Sharma RK, et al. Influence of surgical technique on axillary seroma formation: a randomized study. *ANZ J Surg* 2007;77(5):385–9.
2. Roberts JR, Hedges JR, eds. *Clinical procedures in emergency medicine*, 3rd ed. Philadelphia: WB Saunders, 1998.

10

Permanent Spinal Cord Stimulator Placement

Introduction

Following a successful trial of spinal cord stimulation (SCS), the patient usually wishes to proceed with permanent implantation as soon as possible. The permanent SCS implant poses different challenges than the trial, and these must be considered and planned for in advance. This chapter reviews these issues.

Temporary Versus Permanent Trial

Whether the trial employed a temporary or permanent lead, implanting the permanent system must be scheduled and performed in a fully equipped operating room (OR) with a fluoroscopy table and a C-arm. This is normally an outpatient procedure, after which the patient is discharged with oral analgesics. Before the procedure, the programmer should provide the patient with instructions on how to adjust stimulation, as the patient will likely be too sedated to confirm this ability after the procedure.

Preparation for the permanent system will depend on whether the patient underwent a temporary (percutaneous) or a permanent (tunneled) trial. Each scenario is covered individually.

Permanent Implantation Following a Successful Percutaneous Trial

Before proceeding to a permanent implant after a temporary trial, the small puncture wounds at the entry site of the temporary leads must be adequately healed. The date for a permanent procedure is scheduled when the patient returns to the clinic at the end of a successful trial to have the temporary leads removed. We generally schedule permanent implantation 2 weeks after the conclusion of a successful trial to allow for complete resolution of any residual inflammation at the insertion site of the temporary lead.

The required lead length should be determined before the permanent procedure, as should the need for an extension. A tape measure should be used to measure the distance from the distal end of the trial lead to the prospective site for the implantable pulse generator (IPG). To traverse the distance between the midline and IPG and provide adequate strain relief, it may be necessary to use an extension. The total length of lead required should be known before entering the OR. Implanters who place the IPG in the anterior abdomen often use extensions because of the increased distance to the IPG site. Because strain relief loops have been shown in biomechanical studies to reduce lead tension during lumbar flexion, the lead must be long enough to provide adequate strain relief, both at the anchor and IPG sites.[1] Strain relief is accomplished by coiling loops of lead at the anchor and IPG sites to reduce the risk of lead displacement when the patient bends, stretches, or performs activities causing elongation between the anchor and IPG.

How Much Additional Length Should Be Added for Strain Relief?

There is limited research on which to base a recommendation. A computer modeling study analyzed the effect of spine flexion on the distance between an IPG implanted in the buttock and the midline anchor. In this study, spine flexion caused an increase in distance of 9 cm between the IPG and the anchor.[2] Based on this study, it seems reasonable to recommend that at least one coil of lead or an extension at least 3 cm in diameter (approximately 10 cm of extra length per coil) be placed at the midline and the IPG site for strain relief. This may reduce lead tension during spine flexion and can possibly reduce migration. When it comes to strain relief, too much is better than too little, so it is better to err on the side of overestimation when determining the required length of lead. The strain relief loops should be no smaller than 2.5 cm (1 inch) in diameter to prevent kinking and/or damage to the leads.

Permanent leads often can be tunneled directly without the use of extensions when IPGs are placed in the gluteal region for lumbar SCS or in the axillary region for cervical SCS.

Relevant anatomy of the epidural space, loss of resistance, and fluoroscopic guidance are covered in Chapter 6.

Anesthesia

To ensure proper positioning of the leads, the patient must be alert and communicative during lead placement and intraoperative stimulation testing. Lead placement and anchoring should be performed using local anesthesia with only minimal use of sedation. To reduce the risk of local anesthetic toxicity, we recommend injecting 1% lidocaine with epinephrine, 1:200,000 (methylparaben-free). As much as 7 mg/kg of lidocaine mixed with epinephrine (42 mL in a 60-kg adult) may be injected subcutaneously with minimal risk of toxicity. In the event of an inadvertent intravascular injection, lidocaine also has less cardiotoxicity than bupivacaine.

An anesthesiologist or anesthetist will usually be in charge of monitoring and sedating the patient during permanent SCS placement surgery. Before the surgery, the implanter and anesthesia provider must discuss the different phases of the procedure and agree on the varying sedation requirements necessary for each. Sedation must be minimized during the initial phase of implantation to ensure that the patient is not continually falling asleep and jerking awake during lead positioning and testing. Once the leads have been anchored, heavier sedation can be provided if deemed necessary.

Anterograde Permanent Lead Placement at the Lumbar, Thoracic, and Cervical Levels

Creating the Midline Pocket Incision

The midline incision and undermining process can be performed before or after the leads are placed. These two options are addressed separately below.

Placing the Leads Prior to Cut-Down Incision and Midline Pocket Creation

The advantage of placing the leads prior to the cut-down incision and pocket creation is the ease of moving to a new interlaminar space if needed without having to extend an incision or create a new incision on the opposite side.

The main disadvantage is that making the incision around the placed Tuohy needles is technically more difficult and the dissection may take a bit longer. It is recommended that bipolar electrocautery be used when dissecting around the Tuohy needle to reduce the likelihood of conducting cauterizing electricity into the epidural space.

When placing the Tuohy needle and leads prior to making the cut-down incision, the initial steps involved in patient positioning, needle placement, and lead manipulation for the

permanent procedure are the same as for the percutaneous trial. Please refer to Chapter 7 for more details.

Operative Procedure

As previously discussed, the leads for the permanent implant must be long enough to reach the IPG and allow for adequate strain relief. We commonly use 70-cm leads and, if possible, tunnel directly to the IPG without extensions to reduce the number of electrical connections and any tethering effect of the extension connector.

Choosing Incision Location

At this point, depending on whether one or two leads have been implanted in the epidural space, there are several possible locations for placing the skin incision to create the midline pocket. This stage of the procedure is identical to the procedure for the tunneled trial. Please refer to Chapter 8 for details on this procedure.

Placing the Midline Pocket Cut-Down Incision Prior to Lead Placement

The first advantage to placing the incision prior to lead placement is the time-savings factor, as no dissection is needed around a Tuohy needle. Second, no electrocautery is required until after the Tuohy needles have been removed and the leads are securely anchored. Thus, the use of bipolar electrocautery is usually not necessary.

Although unusual, the major disadvantage to this procedure occurs if fibrosis or some other obstruction is encountered, making entry into a specific interspace problematic or even impossible. If placing the leads at the planned interlaminar space proves impossible, the incision will need to be extended either cephalad or caudad or a second incision on the opposite side of the midline will need to be made. This maneuver is not trivial, as an extended incision or a second unnecessary incision increases postoperative pain and discomfort and produces a suboptimal cosmetic result. For this reason, we do not create a midline pocket prior to lead placement.

Creating the Central Pocket

Please refer to Chapter 8 for details on creating a central pocket.

Anchoring the Lead

Please refer to Chapter 8 for details on anchoring leads.

Permanent Implantation Following Successful Tunneled Trial

Permanent tunneled trials are traditionally performed in a conventional OR (see Chapter 8). If the trial is considered a failure, the patient will return to the OR for lead explantation. If the trial is considered a success, the patient will return to the OR for removal of the temporary extension and implantation of the battery.

Explantation of Temporary Extension

Extensions that are implanted for a temporary trial must be removed to implant the permanent system. In this situation, the extension exit site is under the drape and outside the sterile field. After preparation and draping, the midline pocket is reopened and the extension connector is disconnected from the lead. The extension connector within the pocket is cut with a wire cutter and the remaining extension wire is then pulled out through the exit site from under the drapes by an assistant.

Where to Place the IPG Pocket

The decision as to proper placement of the IPG is controversial and the literature is replete with conflicting expert recommendations. The recommendations of an expert panel based on biomechanical testing results were published in 2006.[2] Based on the results of biomechanical and computer modeling, the panel recommended that IPGs be placed in the abdomen (for lumbar placement) or midaxillary line (for cervical lead placement). Panel members argued that placing the IPG in the buttock region could produce as much as a five-fold increase in lead tension compared with abdominal and midaxillary placement. This recommendation has been contested both in the literature and privately among implanters.[3] Many implanters have successfully placed numerous IPGs in the lateral, lower lumbar area below the belt line and have not

encountered early or late complications such as lead migration or equipment malfunction. One publication notes that abdominal IPG placement in thin patients can result in pressure sores, rib discomfort, pain, and cosmetic dissatisfaction.[4] Subfascial implantation, as recommended in that publication, may be impossible as it could place the IPG too deep for optimal recharging.

We believe that paying strict attention to the anchoring technique and providing adequate strain relief are indispensable in contributing to good long-term outcomes no matter where the IPG is placed. All of us involved in the field of neuromodulation would like to see more clinical studies performed because individual implanters (even the experts) develop diverse preferences and anecdotal opinions that are not evidence-based.

Implanting the IPG in the gluteal region, lateral hip, or buttock below the belt line may be performed with the patient in the prone position. Some implanters tunnel cervical leads with extensions all the way to the upper buttock region and anecdotally claim to have good results. Many, if not most, implanters use the upper gluteal region to implant IPGs for lumbar lead placement. One case study describes a technique for placing the IPG in the superior outer quadrant of the buttock 2 cm inferior and parallel to the inferior rim of the posterior iliac crest.[1] We have used this location successfully with some adjustments depending on where the patient wears a belt (Fig. 10.1).

Placing IPGs in the abdomen or midaxillary line (at the bra line in females) requires that the implant be performed in two stages. First, the patient is prepared and draped in the prone position, with the lead implanted, anchored, and curled within the midline pocket. The wound is then stapled closed and a clear occlusive dressing is placed over the staples. The patient

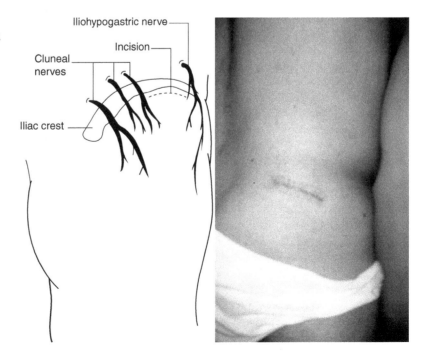

Figure 10.1 Placement of the IPG. Reprinted with permission from Andaluz N, Taha JM. Implantation of the synergy pulse generator in the gluteal area: surgical technique. *Neuromodulation.* 2002;5(2): 72–74. With permission from Wiley-Blackwell.

Iliohypogastric nerve

Incision

Cluneal nerves

Iliac crest

is then turned into the decubitus position, reprepped, and redraped. The occlusive dressing and staples are removed and the midline incision is reopened. Then the abdominal or midaxillary pocket is created and the procedure is completed.

We suggest allowing the patient to choose the location for the IPG site, after being fully informed of the risks and benefits of each option. For some patients the placement of incisions can be an important detail. An implanter should feel comfortable and prepared to vary the IPG location based on a number of factors and be willing to perform the implant in two phases if the patient selects the midaxillary line or abdominal site for the IPG.

For low thoracic lead placement, the pocket for the IPG is most commonly placed in the posterior gluteal area (back pocket), lateral lower lumbar region, mid-flank, or anteriorly in the abdomen inferior to the rib cage. We prefer the outer gluteal region below the belt line. For upper thoracic or cervical placement, the IPG can be placed in the midaxillary region (at the bra line in females or at an analogous level in males) or the supraclavicular region, or even tunneled down to the gluteal region. We prefer the midaxillary location.

Placing the IPG

Proper placement of the IPG should be a decision made before beginning the procedure. The site should be marked with an indelible pen in the preoperative area so that it will still be visible after surgical preparation. If the IPG is being placed in the gluteal region, the patient should wear pants into the preoperative area and a model of the IPG should be placed over the skin with the patient sitting as well as standing so that the proposed pocket site is below the belt line and yet high enough so that the patient will not sit or lie on the unit.

The same procedure should be repeated for midaxillary placement. Female patients should wear a bra in the preoperative area and the site should be marked under the bra line. It is helpful to trace around the model IPG so the pocket location may be precisely identified.

Most rechargeable IPGs should be implanted to a depth of no greater than 2 to 2.5 cm (approximately 1 inch), depending on the manufacturer. It is important that the battery is not implanted too deeply, as it will not recharge properly.

The incision should not overlie the battery. This is especially important when implanting a rechargeable battery. The pocket should be dissected and created inferior to the incision so that the superior edge of the battery is just inferior to the incision when placed into the pocket. This can be accomplished using blunt dissection as described in Chapter 9. The goal is to create a pocket that matches—as precisely as possible—the size of the IPG to reduce dead space. Because the opening of the incision may be slightly stretched to accommodate IPG placement, the length of the incision should be slightly smaller than the diameter of the battery being implanted. This may be as small as 4 cm, which is slightly smaller than the diameter of some of the newer IPGs. Use an IPG template if available or the IPG itself to affirm that the

pocket will accommodate the IPG. Remove the template/IPG and inspect the pocket for bleeders using an Army–Navy retractor. Fulgurate any bleeders using the "cut" mode of a unipolar electrode, or use a bipolar unit.

The Tunneling Procedure – This Procedure Is Detailed in Chapters 8 And 9 but Is Included Again Here for Ease of Reference.

Once the IPG pocket has been created, it is necessary to tunnel the leads from the midline anchor pocket to the IPG pocket. A tunneling tool (Fig. 10.2) is required to pass the lead subcutaneously from the midline lead anchor site to the IPG pocket. A tunneling tool is a sharp-tipped malleable metal shaft that can be bent to conform to the shape of the patient's body. A metal shaft is inserted through a clear plastic cannula sleeve, similar to a straw. Most tunneling tools are manufactured with the plastic cannula preassembled. If not preassembled, the tunneling tool is prepared by slipping the straw over the shaft and screwing the metal handle onto the metal shaft. Tunneling tools are packaged straight, without any bend at the distal tip. It is important that a 10- to 30-degree bend is placed at the distal third of the tunneling tool, depending on the curvature of the patient's anatomy. A curve makes it possible to direct the tip and maintain a superficial depth in the subcutaneous tissue. A firm table should be used for support when bending the tip of the shaft. The tip is sharp and may puncture or cut the surgeon if care is not exercised during bending. The cannula-type tunneling tool may be advanced from midline to the IPG or vice versa. If the distance between the two pockets exceeds the length of the tunneling tool, tunneling will be accomplished in two steps (Fig. 10.3).

Sedation should be increased during the tunneling procedure to reduce the patient's discomfort, and local anesthesia should be administered along the tunneling route. The tunneling unit is advanced through subcutaneous tissue by application of steady force with the dominant hand. It is important

Figure 10.2 Tunneling tools.

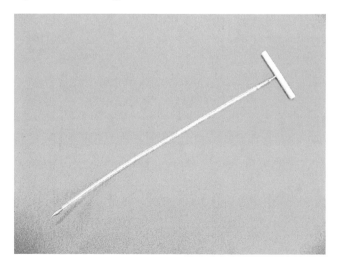

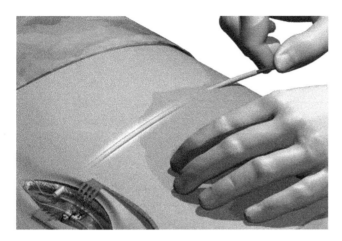

Figure 10.3 Advancement of the tunneling tool.

that the tip of the tunneling tool be felt under the skin with the nondominant hand to gauge depth, and to ensure that the tip is not too deep. The surgeon must confirm that the tool is always in the subcutaneous tissue. If depth and directional adjustments are required, the implanter should steer with the bent tip. Vital structures may be perforated during tunneling if depth is not continuously monitored. The tunneling tool may be passed subcutaneously from the midline incision to the IPG site or vice versa, and the handle is then removed from the tunneling rod, leaving the straw in place. The leads are then inserted through the straw, and the straw is removed through the IPG site. The ends of the leads should be wiped clean with sterile water rather than saline to prevent corrosion and then inserted into the IPG. After the leads have been connected to the IPG and tested successfully, the lead screws on the IPG should be tightened using the torque wrench included

with the device. The wrench should be turned until it clicks several times. The IPG should be placed into the pocket with the letters facing outward toward the skin surface and the extra length of lead looped under the IPG and placed in the midline pocket for strain relief. The strain relief loops should be at least 2.5 cm (1 inch) in diameter to prevent kinking of or damage to the leads. Both midline and IPG incisions should be irrigated generously and closed according to the wound closure techniques described in Chapter 9.

After the Procedure

After the procedure, the patient should be instructed to minimize bending or flexing for 6 weeks to reduce the chance of lead migration. A prefitted soft cervical collar is used to reduce neck motion after cervical SCS placement. The patient is discharged after final programming and asked to engage in minimal activity for the first few days because there will be discomfort at the incision sites once the local anesthetic has worn off.

REFERENCES

1. Kumar K, Hunter G. Spinal epidural abscess. *Neurocrit Care* 2005; 2(3):245–51.
2. Henderson JM, Schade CM, Sasaki J, et al. Prevention of mechanical failures in implanted SCS systems. *Neuromodulation* 2006; 9(3):183–91.
3. Mironer YE. Response to Henderson et al. "Prevention of mechanical failures in implanted spinal cord stimulation systems." *Neuromodulation* 2007;10(1):82–3.
4. Andaluz N, Taha JM. Implantation of the synergy pulse generator in the gluteal area: surgical technique. *Neuromodulation* 2002; 5(2):72–4.

Appendix 1

Dorsal Column Stimulator Implantation
  Patient's Name

  MR#

  DOB

  Operation Date

  Preprocedural Dx

  Postprocedural Dx

  Name of Procedure: Spinal Cord Stimulator and Pulse Generator Implantation

  Anesthesia: Monitored Anesthesia Care with IV sedation

  Estimated Blood Loss: Minimal

  Urine Output: Not Measured

  IV Fluids:

  Complications:

Consent

The risks, benefits, and options were discussed thoroughly with the patient. The patient's questions were answered. The patient appeared to understand and chose to proceed. Informed consent was obtained.

Procedure

Today's permanent implant followed a successful trial of spinal cord stimulation (SCS) and is therefore the second part of a staged procedure. After obtaining informed consent, a 22-gauge IV heplock was placed in the patient's upper extremity. The patient was given an IV prophylactic antibiotic of (1), infused slowly over 30 minutes prior to the procedure. The site for the implantable pulse generator was marked on the patient in the preoperative area. The patient was taken to the operating suite and placed in the prone position with two pillows under the (2). The anesthesia care provider throughout the procedure provided cardiopulmonary monitoring and sedation. The patient's vital signs were noted to be stable during the procedure. The patient's (3) spine was prepped with Betadine and Chlorhexidine and then draped in the usual sterile fashion.

An anteroposterior fluoroscopic view was obtained to identify and mark the midline position of the (4) spinous processes. The skin was anesthetized with (5). Subsequently a 14-gauge 4-inch Tuohy epidural needle provided in the stimulator lead kit was used to approach the epidural space. Local dissection with a No. 15 scalpel and electrocautery was used as necessary to facilitate access to the paraspinous fascia (6). The entry site was at approximately the level of the (7) vertebral body. The needle was advanced using a paramedian approach, to the (8) of midline at approximately a 45-degree angle. Loss-of-resistance to air was utilized to verify placement in the epidural space. The epidural space was entered at the (9) interspace. A lateral fluoroscopic view was obtained to confirm the position of the tip of the Tuohy needle in the epidural space. Aspiration was negative for heme or cerebrospinal fluid. The patient (10) complained of pain or paresthesias during the needle placement. The stylette was removed from the Tuohy needle and the SCS lead was advanced through the Tuohy needle under direct visualization, medially and slightly to the (11) side of midline. The tip of the lead was aligned with the inferior endplate of the (12) vertebral body and was located approximately (13) mm from midline. At this point, a temporary extension was connected to the end of the SCS lead. Stimulator testing was performed with the assistance of the SCS device representative using a temporary extension. The patient reported a (14) pattern of capture covering the (15) at an acceptable voltage. The final position of the zero electrode was noted to be (16) from its previous position. A second lead (17) placed. Following final confirmation of correct lead placement, the midline pocket was fully developed using electrocautery and blunt dissection. Following completion of the midline pocket, the stylette was then removed from the lead followed by the Tuohy needle. When both were removed, the position was rechecked to confirm the lead position had not changed. Stimulation was also rechecked to verify a continued good pattern of capture, and at that point the stimulation (**18**) was anchored to the (**19**) with four 2-0 silk sutures.

The pocket site for the neurostimulator pulse generator was previously identified and marked in the (**20**). (**21**) was used for skin infiltration. Using a No. 15 scalpel, a 4-cm incision was created. A subcutaneous pocket at a depth of approximately 1 to 2 cm was created using blunt dissection. Local anesthetic was then utilized to anesthetize the tract for creating a subcutaneous tunnel between the stimulating lead and the pocket. Using the tunneling tool, tunneling was successfully completed between the midline at the exit site of the lead and the pocket. The lead was then passed through the tunneling tool to the pocket. The lead(s) were then securely placed into the pulse generator and tested. Following successful testing the leads were secured into the pulse generator by tightening the set screws. The pulse generator was then placed into the pocket with the noninsulated lettered side of the unit facing out toward the skin.

At this point, the system was again tested with the pulse generator placed into the subcutaneous pocket. Once the system's function was verified, both the incision sites were irrigated with Bacitracin and closed with 3-0 absorbable multifilament suture. Subcutaneous suturing was accomplished with 4-0 absorbable monofilament suture and cyanoacrylate skin adhesive, followed by the application of Steri-Strips. The wound was then bandaged with sterile gauze and taped down in a sterile fashion.

Initial Stimulator settings: (**24**)

The patient was then brought to the recovery room, where the unit was again tested and activated.

Disposition

The patient was instructed not to reach overhead or perform any abrupt movements with the back, neck, or arms. The patient has been scheduled to return to the pain clinic for follow-up and wound check in approximately 5 days. The patient is to contact the on-call physician on the pain service at any time if there are any complications including, but not limited to, bleeding or signs of infection. There were (**25**) complications. The patient (**26**) tolerated the procedure well and was discharged (**27**) after meeting discharge criteria. At the point of discharge, analgesics were prescribed for home (**28**).

Template

1. Antibiotic given:
   a. 1 g of Kefzol, mixed in 500 cc of normal saline
   b. Other—describe
2. Location of pillows (to reduce lordosis):
   a. Chest to reduce the cervical lordosis
   b. Abdomen to reduce the lumbar lordosis
3. Location of preparation:
   a. Cervical, thoracic, and lumbosacral
   b. Thoracic and lumbosacral
   c. Other—describe
4. Fluoro identification:
   a. C4–T4
   b. T10–L2
5. Local anesthesia:
   a. 1% lidocaine MPF with 1/200,000 epinephrine
   b. Other
6. Local dissection:
   a. Before placement of the Tuohy needle
   b. After placement of the Tuohy needle
7. Skin entry level with Tuohy needle:
   a. T2
   b. L2
   c. Other
8. Paramedian:
   a. Right
   b. Left
9. Site of epidural entry:
   a. Specify level
10. Paresthesias or complaints:
    a. Did
    b. Did not
11. Lead placement:
    a. Right
    b. Left
12. Lead tip location:
    a. Specify level
13. Lead distance from midline:
14. Quality of stim capture:
    a. Good
    b. Fair
    c. Poor, despite multiple attempts at repositioning the lead. Therefore, the stimulator lead and Tuohy needle were completely removed.
15. Upper versus lower extremity or upper versus low back (axial) capture:
    a. Specify location of stim capture
    b. "SKIP" IF NO CAPTURE AND SCS FAILED
16. Final lead position:
    a. Unchanged
    b. Changed (dictate specifics of change in lead position)
    c. "SKIP" IF NO CAPTURE AND SCS FAILED
17. Second lead:
    a. Was
    b. Was not

Repeat 4–16 if a second lead is placed.

18. One or two leads:
    a. Lead was
    b. Leads were each
19. Fascia anchors:
    a. Cervical paraspinous fascia
    b. Lumbar paraspinous fascia
20. Pocket location:
    a. Right upper buttock
    b. Left upper buttock
    c. Other
21. Local anesthesia for pocket:
    a. 1% lidocaine with 1/200,000 epinephrine
    b. Other
22. One or two leads:
    a. Extension was
    b. Two extensions were
23. One or two leads:
    a. The
    b. Each
24. Dictate initial stimulator settings obtained from the product representative.
25. Complications:
    a. None apparent
    b. The following (describe in detail)
26. Tolerance of procedure:
    a. Did
    b. Did not (describe in detail)
27. Length of stay:
    a. From PACU
    b. Following a 23-hour stay
28. Additional recommendations:
    a. Skip
    b. Describe in detail

Postoperative Instructions for Patients Having Spinal Stimulator Implants, Revisions, and Explants

1. Immediate Postoperative Period: It is normal to feel dizzy and sleepy for several hours after your operation. Therefore, you should not drive, operate any equipment, sign any important papers, or make any significant decisions until the next day.
2. Diet: Start with clear liquids. Progress to solids over the next 6 hours. You have received pain medication that may make you sick to your stomach. Soups and foods that are easy to digest are best tolerated as you begin to eat (avoid spicy and fatty food). Drink plenty of fluids. Do not drink alcoholic beverages for 24 hours.
3. Activities: Keep to a minimum.
    a. Resting at home is recommended for 72 hours following your procedure.
    b. No twisting, turning, or bending should be attempted during this time.
    c. Call your physician if your pain is not controlled with pain medication.
4. Temperature: Please report any temperature over 100.4° to your physician. Report any redness, swelling, excessive discharge, or foul odor from the wound. If you develop severe headache or marked neck stiffness and rigidity, please call your physician immediately.
5. Care of the Wound/Special Instructions:
    Keep the surgical area and/or bandage clean and dry.
    Showering should not be attempted postoperatively until your physician instructs you to do so. Sponge bathing is acceptable. Keep the dressing or wound area dry at all times.
    Please keep your dressing intact. If you are prescribed a neck collar or abdominal binder, wear them as instructed by your physician. Change dressing only if/or instructed by your physician.
    For patients with functioning stimulators, spinal cord stimulation may be variable and may change with position. Do not be alarmed! Your unit has a high degree of reliability and usually only minor adjustments are needed. If adjustment is not satisfactory with your hand-held programmer, please contact our office at (xxx) xxx-xxxx.
    You may require modification in your pain medication for immediate postoperative discomfort. Please discuss this with your physician and make changes only as your physician advises.
6. Possible Problems: Report any neurological changes, such as new numbness or weakness or unusually severe back pain. New changes are never normal and may require emergency treatment. If you have any questions or are concerned that something isn't right, please feel free to call our office. If you feel that you are having a true emergency, you must report immediately to an emergency room and the emergency room physician will contact the On-Call Pain Physician directly.

For phone calls after hours: (xxx) xxx-xxxx; ask for a Pain Physician On-Call.

Call the Clinic between 8 am and 5 pm, Monday through Friday, telephone (xxx) xxx-xxxx for an appointment with Dr._____, for _____ (day). Please keep a diary noting your pain responses and side effects every few days until your follow-up visit. Write it down so that you don't forget. Bring the diary with you to your next meeting with your physician.

These instructions have been explained to me. I understand them and have received a copy.

Signature of patient/caretaker:_____

Date:_____ Interpreter:_____

Nurse:_____, R.N.

Sample Preoperative Orders: Spinal Cord Stimulator Implant

Date	Hour	Order
		1. Admit to ambulatory surgical center
		2. Dx: Chronic intractable pain
		3. Patient weight _____
		4. NPO except po/pre-op meds w/H$_2$O sip—after cleared with anesthesia
		5. Start peripheral IV per anesthesia
		6. Notify Dr. XXXXX that patient has arrived
		7. Start Ancef X g IVPB. If allergic to penicillin or cephalosporins, notify surgeon prior to admin.
		8. Void on call to OR

_____

Ordering Physician Signature_____

P.I. #_____Beeper:_____

Nurse/Ancillary Stamp

Sample Preference Card

Site XXX	Pain Service

Double Gloves: 8½ green under 8 regular

Spinal Cord Stimulation/ Dorsal Column

Tape Door Closed with Sign on Door

"No Entry—Implant in Progress"

Positioning/Positioning Supplies

- Prone
- Fluoroscopy table
- Pillows ×4
- Eggcrate mattress
- Elbow foam

PREPARATION
Betadine followed by Hibiclens: Neck to mid-buttock, side to side

INSTRUMENTS
General minor tray

#15 blade

Weitlaner retractor

SUPPLIES
Basic pack

Bar drape ×1

U-drape ×1

10-cc syringe ×2

22-gauge 3½-inch Quincke spinal needle

25-gauge 1½-inch needle

18-gauge 1½-inch needle

Insulated Bovie tip (blade tip)

Bipolar setup

Extra gowns ×2

Ioban drape 6650

Plastic border drapes ×4

C-arm cover

Glass loss-of-resistance

#11 and 15 blades

EQUIPMENT
C-arm (in room before preparation), must print images

Lead aprons and thyroid shields

Spinal cord stimulator lead kit(s) and battery from representative

SUTURES
2-0 silk V-20 ×4

3-0 Polysorb/Vicryl (Popoff) ×12

4-0 Biosyn/Monocryl ×2

Indermil/Dermabond ×2

DRUGS
1% lidocaine MPF w/ epinephrine 1/200,000 30 cc ×2

NaCl irrigation ×2 L mixed with Bacitracin

Bacitracin 100,000 units/L irrigation

DRESSINGS
Half-inch Steri-Strips

Telfa

Medium Tegaderm ×4

Sample Admit and Discharge Orders for Spinal Cord Stimulator 23-Hour Stay

1. Admit to PACU and 23-hour observation
2. Dx: _____
3. Condition: Good
4. VS q shift, neuro checks q 4 hours
5. Allergies: List
6. Activity: Bed rest with bathroom privileges with assistance

7. Keep in:
    a. Abdominal binder
    b. Cervical collar
8. Diet: Regular as tolerated
9. X-ray
    a. PA and lateral thoraco/lumbar
    b. PA and lateral thoraco/lumbar and cervical spine film in PACU
10. Ice pack to incision site(s) for 24 hours
11. Manufacturer representative to instruct patient on stimulator use
12. Analgesic medication examples:
    a. Vicodin 1–2 po q 4 hours prn pain
    b. Percocet 1–2 po q 4 hours prn pain
    c. Dilaudid 0.5–1.0 mg IV q 2 hours prn pain not controlled with above
    d. MSO_4 2–5 mg IV q 10–20 min prn pain not controlled with above
13. Pruritus
    a. Benadryl 25 mg IV q 4–6 hours prn itching
14. IV: Continue present fluids TKO. Use no heparin in patient.
15. Repeat Ancef 1 g IVPB 8 hours following first dose, then 1 g q 8 hours until discharge.
16. Tylenol 1–2 tablets po q 4–6 hours for fever >100°F
17. Reinforce but do not change dressings.
18. Call for:
    a. Temp >100°F
    b. O_2 sat <90, resp rate <10
    c. Extreme somnolence
    d. Numbness, weakness, or new neurological changes
    e. Excessive bleeding or drainage from incision
    f. Excessive pain unrelieved by analgesics ordered

Sample Discharge Orders for Spinal Cord Stimulator 23-Hour Stay

1. Resume normal preoperative medications.
2. Schedule follow-up in pain clinic in 10 days for wound check.
3. Patient may be discharged home after _____ hours of observation if hemodynamically stable, able to void, and having no nausea or uncontrolled pain, following standardized discharge criteria.
4. Sample discharge medications:
    a. Sample pain medications: Vicodin (or Percocet) 1–2 po q 4–6 hours. No. 40

11

Wound Healing, Postoperative Wound Management, and Discharge Education

Introduction

Wound healing is necessary for survival; without it, we would inevitably succumb to hemorrhage and infection. Basic wound-closure techniques describing the use of plant thorns, ant jaws, scalding liquids, and red-hot objects date back thousands of years to the earliest historical records, such as the Smith Papyrus, circa 1700 BC. Although modern tools are more sophisticated, they retain their origins from these primitive thermal and mechanical techniques. Since the discovery of epidermal growth factor in 1962, tremendous advances have occurred in the science of wound care and restoration. The implanter of spinal cord stimulator (SCS) systems must have a basic understanding of wound healing to optimize outcomes and recognize failed or delayed wound healing when it occurs. Many of the same risk factors associated with infection can also affect the process of wound healing.

Normal Wound Healing

Wounded tissue, whether resulting from surgery or other trauma, loses its normal structure and function as the result of external forces. Wound repair is the process whereby the tissue attempts to restore its barriers to fluid loss and infection and increase both blood flow to and structural integrity of the injured region. Normal wound healing proceeds in a predictable sequence that results in functional and structural restoration. Unfortunately, wound healing does not result in regeneration, which is flawless restoration to the preexisting architecture without scar formation. The degree of scar formation and restoration of function depends on the nature of the injury and the quality of the surgical closure. For wound healing to occur, the injured tissue must activate an orderly series of cellular and molecular responses. This process is divided into three phases, as described below (Fig. 11.1).

Phases of Wound Healing

Phase 1: Hemostasis and Inflammation

Hemostasis is the earliest phase of wound healing. Initially, disruption of blood vessels results in transient vasoconstriction, and erythrocytes and platelets serve to initiate hemostasis and plugging of capillaries. Adherence of platelets to capillary endothelium requires the presence of von Willebrand's factor. Platelet activation leads to the release of serotonin and histamine, resulting in vasodilatation and increased permeability of capillaries. Fibrinogen is a soluble plasma protein that extravasates from disrupted vessels and endeavors to seal the rents. Activation of the clotting cascade leads to production of thrombin and formation of fibrin monomers from fibrinogen that polymerize to form clots. The clot matrix allows for the chemotactic attraction of fibroblasts, macrophages, and

Figure 11.1 Phases of wound healing. Reprinted from Mulholland MW. Surgical Complications. In: Townsend CM, Beauchamp RD, Evers BM, et al., eds. *Sabiston textbook of surgery*. Philadelphia: Saunders, 2000. With permission from Elsevier.

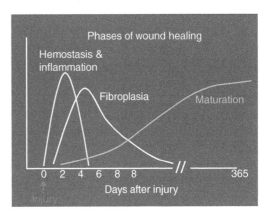

endothelial cells. As fibroblasts begin to produce collagen, the fibrin clot is gradually replaced by scar tissue.

Inflammation begins with the release of complement and chemotactic factors. Monocytes and endothelial cells release inflammatory mediators, such as interleukin-1 and tumor necrosis factor-alpha, which results in movement of neutrophils to the wound site. Nitric oxide has also been shown to play a critical role in the inflammatory response. Nitric oxide signals many biologic processes and is an important metabolite in establishing a defense against invading microorganisms. The clinical findings of redness (rubor), heat (calor), swelling (tumor), and pain (dolor) are consequences of the inflammatory processes resulting from increased vasodilation and capillary permeability.[1]

The inflammatory process peaks between 2 and 4 days post-wound and is characterized by the presence of neutrophils, which are responsible for mopping up wound contaminants, foreign debris, and bacteria.

Circulating monocytes enter the wound next and differentiate into macrophages (Fig. 11.2). Macrophages are critical to wound healing and direct many important processes such as angiogenesis and fibroplasia. Like neutrophils, macrophages also participate in bacterial detection and phagocytosis.

Phase 2: Proliferation and Fibroplasia

It generally takes 3 to 5 days for undifferentiated mesenchymal cells to differentiate into fibroblasts. During this period, known as the "lag phase," the wound is weak and most at risk for dehiscence. The proliferative phase begins with the arrival of fibroblasts at 48 hours and continues over the next several weeks. During this process new blood vessels are formed (angiogenesis), collagen is laid down (fibroplasia), and epithelial resurfacing occurs (epithelialization). Fibroblasts from the surrounding tissue replace the fibrin clot matrix with a loose arrangement of collagen-rich granulation tissue. Proteoglycans and elastins produced by fibroblasts contribute to the integrity of the extracellular granulation tissue. As the number of macrophages decreases, the fibroblast population steadily increases, peaking between 7 and 14 days post-injury. The newly laid collagen begins to contract during this phase, causing the wound edges to be pulled together. Epithelial cells adjacent to

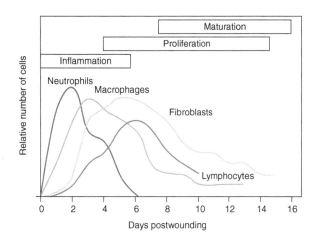

Figure 11.2 Healing time. Reprinted from *Sabiston textbook of surgery*, 17th edition, Figure 8.4. With permission from Elsevier.

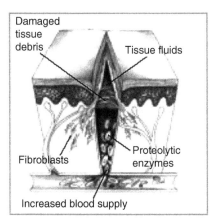

PHASE 1 -
Inflammatory response and debridement process

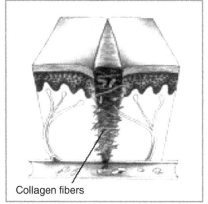

PHASE 2 -
Collagen formation (scar tissue)

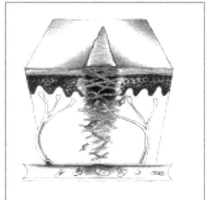

PHASE 3 -
Sufficient collagen laid down

the wound edge begin to proliferate and migrate across the collagen matrix. Of note, epithelial resurfacing of the wound does not contribute to wound strength.

Phase 3: Maturation and Remodeling

The remodeling phase continues over the next 2 years as the wound continues to contract and reorganize. Expression of new collagen results in contraction and increased tensile strength of the wound. During maturation, the fibroblasts in the contracting wound undergo fundamental changes to become more like smooth muscle cells and are referred to as "myofibroblasts." These transformed fibroblasts develop cytoplasmic actin–myosin complexes that greatly accelerate wound contraction. In pathologic states, these transformed fibroblasts contribute to diseases such as hepatic cirrhosis, renal and pulmonary fibrosis, and Dupuytren's contracture. Also, crosslinking of collagen results in further contraction of the wound as it becomes more organized. Even after reorganization has occurred, mature scar tissue is only about 30% to 70% as strong as pristine tissue. Therefore, the SCS implanter should do everything possible to minimize wound size and use optimal surgical and wound-closure techniques to minimize postoperative wound complications.[2]

Identifying the Patient at Risk for Wound Complications

Local and systemic factors can affect wound healing. Complicated healing most often results from bacterial wound contamination. Appropriate preoperative preparation and an aseptic surgical field have been shown to significantly reduce the risk of infection. Please refer to Chapter 4 for more information on sterile surgical techniques. Proper nutrition and overall health factors also affect the rate of wound healing.

Malnutrition, Chronic Disease, and Immune Compromise

Abundant evidence suggests that poor nutritional status and/or immune compromise can influence wound healing and reduce scar tensile strength, predisposing the wound to dehiscence and infection.

Patients with renal disease, diabetes, cancer in remission, or chronic illnesses may have suppressed immune responses, putting them at increased risk for postoperative wound complications. Patients with poor nutritional status—such as malabsorption secondary to gastric bypass or other chronic illnesses such as rheumatoid arthritis, lupus, or HIV—also have compromised immune systems that can influence wound healing. Smoking may also adversely affect wound healing and increase the risk of infection. (Please refer to Chapter 2 for more information on pretrial considerations.)

Patients with diabetes who also have peripheral neuropathy often respond well to SCS. However, they should be under optimal glycemic control before proceeding with a trial. Elevated blood glucose levels in the postoperative period predispose patients to infection and delayed wound healing. This results, at least in part, from interference with chemotaxis of phagocytosis and delayed leukocyte and macrophage migration. The result is a prolonged inflammatory phase.

Patients with any chronic illness should be medically and nutritionally optimized to the greatest extent possible. Optimizing the patient's nutritional status with the aid of a dietitian or nutritional consultant can contribute to an uncomplicated postoperative course.[3] Our philosophy is to medically optimize our patients before proceeding with implantation surgery. Fortunately, relative to other more invasive surgeries, SCS implantation results in a modest physiologic stress response.

Postoperative Care

Most patients are discharged on the same day as their surgery. Resting at home is recommended for at least the first 2 postoperative days. Pain, discomfort, and swelling normally peak on postoperative day 2 and should begin to decrease after that. Adequate pain medication in addition to the patient's usual chronic pain medication is prescribed. The patient is advised to avoid sudden movements, bending, lifting, stretching, reaching, pulling, or twisting for the first 4 to 6 weeks.

Showering

There has been insufficient research to determine the amount of time needed before patients can safely begin showering postoperatively. Conventional instruction has been to keep the wound clean and dry for 10 to 14 days or until 1 to 2 days after suture or staple removal. Although there is some difference of opinion, most seem to agree that the wound should be kept completely dry for at least the first 48 hours postoperatively. Some implanters who use adhesives to close the wound, such as Dermabond or Indermil, would argue that because the wound is "sealed" the patient should be able to shower immediately after the procedure. A prospective study analyzed the effect of showering between 2 and 5 days after posterior spine surgery in patients with stapled wounds. The investigators found no increase in wound complications in the group that showered.[4] Another prospective study in Finland also found no difference in wound complications in patients following herniorrhaphy who used saunas beginning on postoperative day 3.[5] Because we use absorbable suture and wound adhesives for closure, we allow our patients to shower after the first wound check on postoperative day 3 if the wound appears normal.

At the first postoperative wound check, the dressings should be removed and the wound(s) inspected and gently cleaned with peroxide and a cotton-tipped swab. Sterile gloves should be worn while palpating for areas of tenderness or fluctuance. It is common to see a 2- to 3-mm rim of redness around the wound edge; however, this area of redness should not spread. If a surgical site infection is suspected, baseline laboratory studies should be obtained, including a complete blood count, sedimentation rate, and C-reactive protein. Increases in pain, swelling, or redness and the presence of fever, chills, or drainage from the wound after the first postoperative wound check should be thoroughly evaluated. A tissue ultrasound can be helpful in differentiating seroma from infection. Patients with questions should be seen in the office the next day for a follow-up wound check. (See Chapter 12 for more information on complications and infection.) Evidence of expanding erythema or increases in tenderness should be treated as infection until proven otherwise.

Postoperative Antibiotics

Use of prophylactic postoperative antibiotics is controversial. There is no evidence to suggest that they decrease the rate of wound infection beyond that of initial preoperative antibiotic administration. Administering postoperative antibiotics also poses the risk of selecting out resistant organisms, which may make treating a surgical site infection more problematic.

Suture and/or Staple Removal

Nonabsorbable skin sutures or staples should be removed between postoperative days 7 and 10. This can usually be performed on the second postoperative visit.

1. First postoperative wound check at postoperative day 3 or 4
   a. Remove outer dressing but leave Steri-Strips intact if present. Loose Steri-Strips may be removed. It is not necessary to redress the remaining Steri-Strips or replace those removed as they will fall off by themselves. Loose material should be gently cleaned away with peroxide. A 4 × 4 gauze pad should be placed over the wound(s) and taped loosely. The patient may shower if the wound shows no sign of infection. The surgical site may be patted dry but should not be vigorously rubbed with a towel.
   b. No bathing or soaking
2. Second postoperative wound check between postoperative days 7 and 10
   a. If present, staples and/or nonabsorbable sutures should be removed.
   b. No bathing or soaking
3. Final postoperative wound check at 3 weeks
   a. If the wound shows no sign of infection, the patient may now bathe or soak.

REFERENCES

1. Mulholland MW. Surgical complications. In Townsend CM, Beauchamp RD, Evers BM, et al., eds. *Sabiston textbook of surgery*. Philadelphia: Saunders, 2000.
2. Hollinsky C, Sandberg S. Measurement of the tensile strength of the ventral abdominal wall in comparison with scar tissue. *Clin Biomech* 2007;22:88–92.
3. Collins N. Diabetes, nutrition, and wound healing. *Adv Skin Wound Care* 2003;16(6):291–4.
4. Carragee EJ, Vittum DW. Wound care after posterior spinal surgery: does early bathing affect the rate of wound complications? *Spine* 1996;21(18):2160–2.
5. Papp AA, Alhava EM. Sauna-bathing with sutures: a prospective and randomised study. *Scand J Surg* 2003;92(2):175–7.

12

Complications and Adverse Events

"In surgery, a surgeon's experience can be measured by his complications, but his wisdom is measured by how he deals with it."

William S. Halstead

Postoperative Complications in the Modern World

Surgery entails certain risks, and complications are inevitable. It has been said that given enough cases, every conceivable surgical complication will occur to someone, somewhere, at some point. In the past, the subject of complications was a matter limited to discussion between the patient and surgeon. The surgeon generally handled common postoperative complications, such as infections, without running the risk of malpractice or litigation. In fact, a surgeon could even have a high complication rate without suffering any negative consequences. This, however, is no longer the case.

Hospital quality improvement committees, and society at large, now track and scrutinize information that was formerly confidential and private between the patient and surgeon. Complication rates for individual hospitals are now public record and available to patients via the Internet. Benchmarks have been established and evidence-based standards are used by accreditation and oversight agencies to rank hospitals based on predetermined quality indicators. Data on individual surgeons may also be in the public domain. Patients have become informed consumers and demand assurance that they are getting the best care available. It is now possible for patients to choose their provider based on comparative aggregate outcome data. Seniority and experience are becoming less important in the age of real-time outcome tracking. Furthermore, insurance companies are beginning to link reimbursement rates with outcomes, a "pay-for-performance" policy. In 2000, the Institute of Medicine published a scathing report entitled "To Err Is Human: Building a Safer Health System," which noted that 44,000 to 98,000 people die each year from preventable medical errors.[1]

Implantation of analgesic devices is part of this evolving picture, and future implanters must be prepared to avoid complications whenever possible and know how to manage complications that do arise.

Training

At a time when information technology is rapidly expanding, it is nearly impossible for anyone to keep up with every advance in surgical practice. The exponential increase in published studies in every field and the increasing complexity of basic and clinical research present tremendous challenges for modern practitioners. The quality of individual training and the knowledge of institutional policies are critical, as both affect clinical outcomes. Complication rates can vary significantly by individual and institution and are not the result of random chance or "a string of bad luck." These rates can be significantly affected by changes in practice and policies. A recent publication by the American Health Quality Association demonstrated how 56 hospitals in Washington, Alaska, and Idaho collaborated and adopted protocols that reduced surgical infection rates by 27% per year.[2]

Implanting spinal cord stimulators (SCSs) requires advanced training and seasoned clinical judgment. Attending a weekend cadaver course (or simply reading a book, including this one) does not provide adequate training. It would obviously be a concern if a practitioner with inadequate training was encouraged to begin performing procedures, as this could result in significant harm not only to the patient, but also to the clinician and facility involved. All future implanters must be appropriately trained in all areas relevant to SCS systems. The specifics of training may vary but in almost all cases should involve direct work with a mentor over an extended period of time, supplemented by didactic self-learning tools (e.g., written and video educational materials) as well as cadaver workshops. This book serves as part of such a training program. Formal training in a program accredited by the Accreditation Council on Graduate Medical Education is the gold standard.

Complications and Adverse Events

The first thing a training implanter must learn is not to be a hero. If an unfamiliar complication arises, help should be sought. Complications associated with SCS are divided into three categories: anesthetic, surgical, and hardware complications (Table 12.1).

The most common surgical complications are infection (5%), wound hematoma, and seroma.[3] In a 1995 meta-analysis summarized by Stojanovic and Abdi, the most common hardware complications were lead migration (24%), lead failure (7%), and pulse generator failure (2%) (Table 12.2).[3–5] Advances in technology, protocols, and experience in SCS implantation have likely reduced these rates today.

Anesthesia Complications

Monitoring

Patients should be constantly monitored for hemodynamic stability during SCS trials and permanent implants. At a minimum, pulse oximetry, blood pressure monitoring with an automated cuff, and electrocardiography should be routine in all cases. Supplemental nasal cannula oxygen should be administered at 2 to 4 L per minute.

The standards of the American Society of Anesthesiologists (ASA) mandate the following:[6]

1. Personnel trained to provide sedation and monitor vital signs, including respirations, must be present and monitor the patient constantly throughout the procedure.

Table 12.1

Adverse Events Associated with SCS

- Anesthetic complications
  - Poor monitoring
  - Local anesthetic toxicity
  - Inadvertent subarachnoid injection
- Surgical complications
  - Infection
  - Hematoma
  - Seroma
  - Dural punctures and cerebrospinal fluid hygromas
  - Dehiscence
  - Perforated viscus—tunneling
  - Cord injury and nerve damage
  - Sedation
  - Stenosis
- Hardware complications
  - Lead fracture and migrations

Table 12.2

The Most Common Complications of SCS Leads in Two Studies

Complication	Incidence (%)	Prevention and Treatment
Lead migration	12.3–13.2	Anchor the lead properly, strain relief
Lead breakage	6.8–9.1	Insert anchor through fascia
Infection	3.3–3.4	Follow sterile procedures
Poor coverage	12.3	Reprogram unit

2. Continuous monitoring must be performed with pulse oximetry, continuous electrocardiography, and regular intermittent blood pressure monitoring. Additional monitoring is required during general anesthesia.

Local Anesthetic Toxicity

SCS trials and permanent implants are generally performed with local anesthesia (LA) and light to moderate sedation. Sedation should be light during lead placement as outlined in previous chapters. Considerable volumes of LA are often required during permanent implantation to maintain patient comfort. The risk of developing LA toxicity is real and may be increased in patients with renal or hepatic dysfunction, chronic obstructive pulmonary disease with respiratory acidosis, pre-existing heart conditions and heart block, and extreme age. The most common cause of toxicity is inadvertent intravascular injection.

The most effective means of managing LA toxicity is to prevent it. The total dose (mg/kg) of LA that can safely be administered should be calculated and care taken not to exceed it. Aspiration should be performed before LA injection to ensure the needle is not intravascular or intrathecal. Doses should be delivered in incremental units so accidental intravascular injections can be recognized before a large volume is administered.

The risk of LA toxicity can be reduced by injecting the skin and the planned path of the needle with 1% lidocaine with epinephrine, 1:200,000 (methylparaben-free). As much as 7 mg/kg of lidocaine mixed with epinephrine (42 mL for a 60-kg adult) can be injected subcutaneously with minimal risk of toxicity. Lidocaine has a short half-life; half the initial dose can therefore be repeated in approximately 1.5 to 2 hours in adult patients who do not have liver impairment, renal disease, or heart failure. In the event of an inadvertent intravascular injection, lidocaine has less cardiotoxicity than bupivacaine.

Early signs of central nervous system (CNS) toxicity from LAs include light-headedness, dizziness, drowsiness, disorientation, shivering, muscle twitching, and tremors in the face and distal extremities. If anesthetic toxicity is suspected, the first priority is to immediately address and stabilize potential life-threatening situations. In cases of inadvertent rapid intravenous (IV) injection, CNS excitation such as seizure activity may rapidly give way to CNS depression, respiratory arrest, and coma. Treating imminent airway compromise, hypotension, and dysrhythmia takes priority over other surgical considerations. If the patient is prone on the operating room table, the wound should immediately be covered with an occlusive dressing, if available, and the patient turned to a supine position onto a gurney. Basic and advanced life support protocols must be initiated immediately according to preexisting guidelines. When the patient is no longer in immediate danger, any additional associated complications such as nausea or dizziness can be treated.

If CNS toxicity or seizures occur, steps must be taken to prevent permanent injury. Intravascular injection of LA usually results in very transient CNS toxicity, whereas toxicity from excessive subcutaneous administration may persist for some time. Seizures from LA toxicity result in a hypermetabolic state that can rapidly lead to hypoxemia, hypercarbia, and acidosis. Resuscitative efforts must be undertaken immediately to prevent permanent hypoxemic injury to the CNS. Immediate initiation of basic life-support strategies can be life saving. The basic ABCs—airway, breathing, and circulation—must be put into action. The airway should be patent and supplemental oxygen should be administered by mask with an Ambu-bag if the patient is not breathing. Intubation is not mandatory if adequate ventilation and sufficient oxygen saturation levels are maintained, but the patient must be intubated immediately if assisted ventilations by mask are inadequate. Administration of midazolam or other available benzodiazepines can help control seizure activity in the patient with stable vital signs. It may take several minutes to achieve seizure control after administration. Barbiturates and IV propofol have also been shown to control anesthetic-induced seizures and muscle twitching, although these drugs are often not available in office-based procedure rooms, where many trials are performed. Use of phenytoin (Dilantin) should be avoided because its sodium channel-blocking effects may potentiate LA toxicity.

Overt cardiac toxicity is usually not seen with lidocaine administration because the threshold for neurotoxicity is significantly lower than that for cardiotoxicity. This is not the case with bupivacaine. Although bupivacaine has advantages because of its longer half-life, toxicity can be life-threatening. Cardiovascular toxicity may be preceded by prolongation of PR, QRS, and QT intervals as a precursor to aberrant conduction. In such cases, class IB antiarrhythmic agents such as mexiletine (Mexitil) and tocainide (Tonocard) must be avoided because their sodium channel-blocking properties may potentiate LA cardiac toxicity.

Impaired ventricular contractility results from inhibition of calcium, potassium, and sodium channels, leading to conduction blockade and cardiac dysrhythmias that are often refractory to intervention. Loss of peripheral vascular tone makes chest compressions less effective at generating effective cerebral perfusion. In these instances, cardiac resuscitation will be difficult and prolonged (45–60 minutes) because LAs are highly lipid-soluble and require a prolonged period for redistribution. Ventricular tachycardia, fibrillation, and asystole have all been described as secondary to LA toxicity and should be treated according to the Advanced Cardiac Life Support (ACLS) guidelines published by the American Heart Association. Table 12.3 provides a sample treatment protocol that may be used in conjunction with ACLS protocols.

Recent case reports indicate that an infusion of lipid emulsion may be life-saving in some instances. Data supporting the use of lipid emulsion is most encouraging relative to bupivacaine cardiotoxicity. A recent case of refractory cardiac arrest following intravascular injection of bupivacaine was reversed following IV administration of 100 mL of 20% Intralipid.[7] Having Intralipid available, similar to dantrolene for malignant hyperthermia, may become the standard of care when bupivacaine is being administered. The salvific effects of Intralipid may or may not apply to other LAs.

Inadvertent Subarachnoid Injection: The Total Spinal Block

An inadvertent injection of even a small amount of LA into the intrathecal space can result in a spinal block. If a large volume of LA is administered, or an intrathecal injection occurs at the high thoracic level, a high spinal or total spinal block can occur. A high spinal block will result in temporary total paralysis with ventilatory compromise and a complete sympathectomy compounded by profound bradycardia in the face of severe hypotension. A total spinal block will result in loss of consciousness and respiratory arrest. If a large volume of LA has been administered into the subarachnoid space, ventilatory support requiring intubation and manual/mechanical ventilation will be needed for several hours until spontaneous ventilation returns. Initial support of arterial blood pressure and heart rate requires placing the patient in the Trendelenburg position to maximize venous return and administering IV atropine and ephedrine. A more potent

Table 12.3
ACLS Protocol Supplementation

- Begin ACLS resuscitation protocol
  Cardiopulmonary resuscitation may be prolonged (up to 1 hour)
- Intubation
- Fluids
- Vasopressor
  Epinephrine (0.2–0.5 mcg/kg per minute)
  Phenylephrine (0.2–0.75 mcg/kg per minute)
  Norepinephrine (0.02–0.5 mcg/kg per minute)
- Follow ACLS guidelines
  Vasopressin, amiodarone, Mg
  Treat local anesthetic-induced seizures with benzodiazepines, barbiturates (thiopental 2 mg/kg), or propofol (1 mg/kg).
  Avoid phenytoin.
- Low cardiac output states
  Milrinone possibly superior to epinephrine
- Cardiopulmonary bypass if available

ACLS, Advanced Cardiac Life Support.

sympathomimetic infusion, such as epinephrine, should also be prepared. When a large dose of LA is injected into the cerebrospinal fluid (CSF), the patient will lose consciousness and develop dilated pupils. This does not indicate CNS injury, and the pupils will become normal and reactive as the anesthetic block resolves. Because the patient is unconscious during tracheal intubation and mechanical ventilation, sedation requirements are minimal. Fortunately, most patients have no memory of the event after resolution of the block and extubation.[8]

Surgical Complications

Infection

Preoperative Prevention

Patients with active infections are not candidates for SCS implantation. In questionable situations, obtaining a complete blood count (CBC) with differential analysis, urinalysis, and erythrocyte sedimentation rate (ESR) can help identify at-risk patients. Depending on the location and severity of an earlier bacterial infection, implant surgery may be postponed until an antibiotic course is completed and symptoms and laboratory studies have normalized.

Postoperative Infection

Surgical site infections (SSIs) are the bane of the SCS implanter. Infections following surgeries such as joint replacements, cosmetic enhancement procedures, and pacemaker implantations account for about 50% of the 2 million hospital-acquired infections that occur in the United States each year.[9] There is nothing more devastating than having to explant a system that is functioning well and providing excellent pain relief, so every possible measure should be taken to prevent a postoperative infection. Please refer to Chapter 4 for more information on sterile technique.

In a case series of more than 100 patients, the incidence of wound infection (superficial or deep) following SCS implantation was 2% to 5% and the risk of meningitis or epidural abscess was less than 0.5%.[10] The majority of SSIs result from infection with *Staphylococcus* or *Streptococcus*. Resistant strains, such as methicillin-resistant *Staphylococcus aureus,* are becoming more prevalent even in community-acquired cases, making treatment more problematic.

Early diagnosis of an SSI can be difficult because pain and discomfort are common in the immediate postoperative period. When pain begins to increase after a period of improvement, an SSI should be considered. The signs of postoperative inflammation normally begin to diminish after 5 to 7 days. It is during this window, between postoperative days 3 and 5, that signs of acute infection gradually become apparent, although later onset can also occur. It is common at the time of the first postoperative wound check (postoperative day 3)

to see a 2- to 3-mm rim of redness around the wound's edge. However, this area of redness should not expand and increased tenderness should not be present. Increased wound tenderness is usually consistent with early onset of an SSI, although fever is often initially absent. Redness, warmth, and swelling are not specific but may indicate infection. Increases in pain, swelling, or redness and the presence of fever, chills, or drainage from the wound suggest an SSI. Drainage may be absent at first if the wound was sealed with adhesive during surgery.

If an SSI is suspected, baseline laboratory studies, including a CBC, ESR, and C-reactive protein (CRP), should be drawn. However, these laboratory values are nonspecific and can be elevated in the patient without postoperative complications. SCS implantation surgery is minimally traumatic, however, and should not produce the same laboratory value changes associated with more invasive surgeries. The ESR has been shown to peak at postoperative day 5, with a slow decline to normal over the next 30 days. CRP has been shown to peak between postoperative days 2 and 3 after uncomplicated spine surgery, with normalization occurring between postoperative days 5 and 14. Postoperative laboratory values are generally not abnormal in the patient without complications following SCS implantation, but this is anecdotal. An elevated white count with left shift, ESR, and CRP should be taken seriously and repeated to establish a trend.[11] In equivocal cases, ultrasound is sometimes helpful in differentiating seroma from infection. If inconclusive, the patient should undergo an additional wound check the following day. Progressive erythema around the wound or increased tenderness should be treated as an infection until proven otherwise.

There have been documented cases of successful resolution of superficial wound and pocket infections with oral and IV antibiotics without removal of the device. Nonetheless, treating an SSI without removing the SCS device in its entirety poses a risk. SCS leads form a conduit from the superficial midline pocket to the epidural space. This allows infection to spread into the epidural space, resulting in meningitis and epidural abscess.[10] It is recommended that the device be removed in its entirety if an SSI occurs. Cultures should be tested for sensitivity, and broad-spectrum antibiotics that are effective in treating *Staphylococcus* and *Streptococcus* should be initiated empirically. Once the organism is identified and antibiotic sensitivities have been obtained, antibiotic therapy can be modified. Once the device has been removed and the wound irrigated thoroughly, a drain, such as a 7-mm Jackson Pratt, should be placed before closure. If drainage is minimal, the drain can usually be removed in 3 to 4 days.

If the wound infection persists, the wound may need to be left open and allowed to close by secondary intention. Allowing healing by secondary intention is often necessary in infected wounds or burns and occurs via the formation of granulation tissue, which results in eventual coverage of the defect by spontaneous epithelialization. A general surgical consultation may be of value in this situation.[12]

Epidural abscess is also a serious infectious complication that must be considered when the patient complains of pain or other discomfort consistent with infection or has consistent laboratory findings. Epidural abscess is discussed below along with epidural hematoma because the presenting signs, symptoms, and immediate treatment responses are very similar.

Hematoma

Preoperative Prevention

> *"The only weapon with which the unconscious patient can immediately retaliate upon the incompetent surgeon is hemorrhage."*
>
> William S. Halsted

The competent surgeon must take every step possible to avoid such an outcome. To reduce the chance of hemorrhage, the patient should be advised to stop taking any antiplatelet or anticoagulation agents before the procedure. If applicable, use of clopidogrel (Plavix) and aspirin should be discontinued 7 days before surgery and ticlopidine (Ticlid) should be stopped 14 days before surgery. Some surgeons may be willing to implant SCS systems in patients unable to discontinue use of aspirin. However, data are lacking in patients taking aspirin when epidural anesthesia is used. The absence of data demonstrating an increased incidence of epidural hematoma does not necessarily imply absence of risk. The literature continues to report isolated cases of neurologic injury after epidural anesthesia in patients taking antiplatelet drugs. The use of neuraxial techniques, including SCS, in patients taking newer and more potent antiplatelet drugs requires caution and conservative management until adequate clinical trials have been conducted.[8]

SCS implantation in a patient who will be resuming anticoagulation therapy postoperatively is controversial. Although the risk of hematoma is likely small, there are no data to quantify that risk. Epidural hematoma has been documented in patients with no known risk factors for postoperative bleeding.[13] As of August 2007, there were no reports of epidural hematoma after placement of high thoracic epidural catheters before cardiac bypass with anticoagulation. Although this is thought by some to result from underreporting, it is still a remarkable finding.[14] Compared with epidural catheters, SCS leads are stiffer and larger in diameter and can move in the epidural space. Therefore, the risks of SCS lead placement and that of epidural catheters may not be analogous. Unfortunately, there are no data quantifying the risk for epidural hematoma with indwelling leads in either acute or chronic SCS patients who require chronic anticoagulation. Again, the absence of data does not imply an absence of risk. Caution and conservative management are therefore recommended when treating patients taking anticoagulants or platelet inhibitors.

If SCS is indicated in a patient requiring anticoagulation therapy, warfarin should be discontinued 7 days before surgery and low-molecular-weight heparin (LMWH) should be initiated as a bridge. Table 12.4 provides a sample protocol.[15]

An international normalized ratio (INR) should be obtained the day before surgery and the last dose of LMWH should be withheld the day before surgery. By definition, placing epidural leads is a neurosurgical procedure, and the INR should be 1.2 or less. For non-neurosurgical procedures, such as implantable pulse generator (IPG) exchanges, an INR of less than 1.5 is probably safe.

Postoperative Hematoma

The gravity of a postoperative hemorrhage depends on the location and volume of the bleed. An incisional or IPG pocket hematoma can often be managed conservatively, but an epidural hematoma is a surgical emergency.

Epidural Hematoma

A retrospective meta-analysis published in 2001 suggested that the risk of epidural hematoma is approximately 1 in 150,000 following epidural anesthesia.[16] Although rare, a clinically significant epidural hematoma will result in paralysis if not treated immediately. Onset of symptoms can be immediate or

Table 12.4

Sample Protocol for Bridging Coumadin with Low-Molecular-Weight Heparin[15]

Preoperative Protocol
- Stop warfarin 7 days before surgery.
- Start LMWH 36 hours after last warfarin dose; for example: Enoxaparin 1 mg/kg subcutaneously every 12 hours, *or* Enoxaparin 1.5 mg/kg subcutaneously every 24 hours, *or* Dalteparin 120 U/kg subcutaneously every 12 hours, *or* Dalteparin 200 U/kg subcutaneously every 24 hours, *or* Tinzaparin 175 U/kg subcutaneously every 24 hours
- Give last dose of LMWH approximately 24 hours before procedure.
- Educate patient in self-injection or arrange for injections at Coumadin Clinic.
- Discuss plan with anesthesiologist.
- Check that INR is less than 1.2 on the day of surgery if implanting SCS epidural leads, or less than 1.5 if implanting IPG only.

Postoperative Protocol
- Restart LMWH 24 hours after procedure and consider a reduced thromboprophylactic dose (i.e., enoxaparin 0.75 mg/kg subcutaneously every 12 hours) of LMWH on postoperative day 1 after SCS implantation.
- Restart warfarin at patient's previous dose on postoperative day 1.
- Obtain periodic prothrombin time and INR until INR is in the therapeutic range.
- Patient should be followed up on a daily basis by the Coumadin Clinic nurse to assess for adverse effects such as bleeding.
- CBC and platelets should be monitored at the first and second wound check visit.
- Discontinue LMWH when INR is between 2.0 and 3.0 for 2 consecutive days.[15]

CBC, complete blood count; INR, international normalized ratio; IPG, implantable pulse generator; LMWH, low-molecular-weight heparin; SCS, spinal cord stimulation.

delayed from hours to days after placement or removal of an epidural catheter. Thus, maintaining a high index of suspicion is important.[16,17] If a patient develops neurologic symptoms consistent with a neuraxial mass following SCS lead placement, an emergent computed tomography (CT) scan, immediate neurosurgical intervention, and decompression are indicated if permanent paralysis is to be prevented. Early symptoms can vary but may include back pain, radicular pain, progressive weakness, sensory changes (i.e., saddle anesthesia), and incontinence. Lower extremity weakness and incontinence suggest a significant mass resulting in spinal cord compression by the hematoma. Case reports suggest that partial to near-complete neurologic recovery can occur if surgical decompression is accomplished within 8 hours of symptom onset. Performing decompression more than 8 hours after symptom onset invariably results in paralysis.[18]

Epidural Abscess

The signs and symptoms of epidural abscess can be similar to those of epidural hematoma save that their onset is often delayed. Treatment of epidural abscess in patients with implanted SCS systems involves emergent surgical evacuation and explantation of the device, followed by antibiotic therapy. New-onset neurologic deficit, persistent fever, leukocytosis, and severe pain are all strong indications for surgical decompression and explantation.[19] Presenting symptoms vary with the degree of cord compression but include back pain, pain on any Valsalva maneuver (such as during bowel movements), fever, urinary retention, bowel/bladder incontinence, and progressive extremity weakness leading to paraplegia. Spine percussion over the area of the abscess is often exceedingly painful. Reflexes may be hyper- or hypoactive, with positive upper motor neuron signs. Nuchal rigidity can be present in patients with cervical epidural abscesses. If an epidural abscess is suspected, patients with implanted SCSs should have baseline laboratory blood tests performed, including a CBC, ESR, and CRP, and an emergent CT scan.[20] If an epidural abscess is diagnosed in patients with neurologic deficits, emergent surgical decompression and drainage of the abscess along with explantation of the SCS system should be performed.

Hematoma of the Midline or IPG Pocket

A hematoma is a collection of blood that most often occurs in the subcutaneous layer beneath the surgical wound. Hematomas are more worrisome than seromas because of the increased risk of infection. The best treatment for an incisional or pocket hematoma is prevention. Meticulous attention to hemostasis and gentle wound handling before wound closure helps to avoid postoperative problems. The overall incidence of hematoma is low because of the widespread use of electrosurgical hemostasis.

Wound hematomas frequently present with a blue/purple discoloration of the skin overlying the wound. Small low-volume hematomas without significant pain carry a somewhat increased risk of infection because blood is an excellent culture medium, but they will often resorb on their own without

surgical intervention. The risk of reopening the wound exceeds letting a small hematoma resolve on its own. The patient will often have widespread ecchymosis that slowly resorbs over time. On the other hand, a large expanding hematoma within a closed space can be very painful and may progress to wound dehiscence. The patient may not be febrile, but the wound will be swollen, tense, and painful to palpation. Expanding hematomas should be evacuated surgically under sterile conditions.[18,21]

If a clinically significant hematoma is suspected, baseline laboratory blood tests, including a CBC, ESR, and CRP, should be drawn to help rule out infection. An ultrasound can be helpful to differentiate seroma, hematoma, and infection. If an expanding hematoma is left untreated, wound dehiscence and infection can result. A painful expanding hematoma should be surgically evacuated and irrigated thoroughly and the source of bleeding identified. The use of electrosurgical fulguration, either monopolar or bipolar, may damage some IPG units. The manufacturer of the SCS should be consulted to determine whether electrosurgical fulguration is acceptable. If not, a handheld battery-operated disposable electrocautery unit should be used to fulgurate bleeders in wounds with implanted IPGs. An electrocautery unit will heat the tissue but will not pass current through the patient; therefore, no damage will be caused to the IPG (Fig. 12.1). If the hematoma is caught early, the wound can frequently be closed primarily.

Midline or IPG Pocket Seroma

Although seromas are one of the most benign surgical complications, they must be followed closely to ensure they do not develop into infections. A seroma is a collection of serous fluid that forms beneath the wound and does not consist of blood, CSF, or pus. Seromas consist of serum, liquefied fat, and lymphatic fluid. Swelling around the IPG pocket can be caused by seroma, hematoma, hygroma, or infection. These complications can be difficult to distinguish from each other. A large seroma is often painful as a result of compression within a closed space and may increase the risk of infection. Some studies have shown that liberal use of electrocautery dissection can contribute to postoperative seroma. However, a recent prospective randomized study found no difference in the rate of seroma formation whether electrocautery or scissor dissection was used during mastectomy.[22] We use a combination of sharp dissection for the skin incision, followed by careful blunt dissection, and the use of "cut" mode for electrosurgical dissection, as outlined in Chapter 9. Although there are many variations, the common theme should be to minimize tissue trauma and reduce seroma formation while ensuring excellent hemostasis.

The clinical presentation of seroma is similar to that of hematoma. The patient will not be febrile, but the wound may be swollen, tense, and painful to palpation. If a clinically significant seroma is suspected, baseline laboratory blood tests, including a CBC, ESR, and CRP, should be drawn to help rule out infection. An ultrasound can be helpful to differentiate between seroma, hematoma, and infection.

Seromas delay healing and increase the risk of infection. A seroma can be monitored if there is no increased pressure

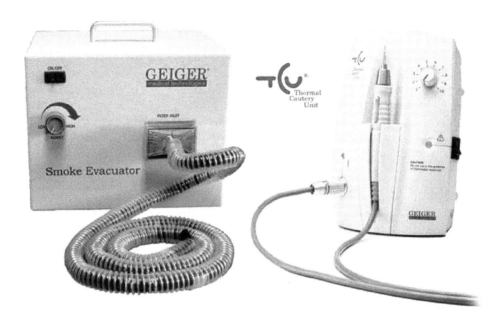

Figure 12.1a,b Electrocautery unit. Reprinted with permission from © 2009 Geiger Medical. All rights reserved.

over the wound and it is not tender. If the seroma is tense and painful, it can be serially aspirated. The area must be aseptically prepared before aspirating to prevent bacteria from entering the wound. We prefer to perform aspirations under fluoroscopy to avoid damaging the SCS leads with the needle. The aspirate should be sent for culture, sensitivity testing, and fluid analysis to rule out infection or presence of CSF. Monitoring of the patient should continue. An abdominal binder can offer a countering force that may facilitate resolution of the seroma. Empirical antibiotics are not recommended for seromas as the entire system must be explanted and IV antibiotics initiated if cultures are positive for bacterial organisms. If a dural puncture occurred during the procedure, the collection at the midline pocket could be CSF (hygroma) and should be managed as described in the next section. Some physicians advocate placing a vacuum drain in refractory cases, although drains themselves can be a source of infection. Most seromas can be managed conservatively with an abdominal binder and if necessary fluoroscopically guided serial aspirations using sterile technique, with each aspirate sample being sent for culture and sensitivity testing.[12,18]

Dural Punctures and CSF Hygromas

Dr. Leonard Corning, a neurologist from New York, was the first to consider the idea of injecting an anesthetic into the subarachnoid space. In 1885, he injected cocaine into a patient's thoracic spine and produced a spinal anesthetic block. In 1889, Drs. August Bier and August Hildebrand performed spinal blocks on each other. The following morning both of them had developed headaches. Dr. Bier described a "strong pressure on my skull and rather dizzy when I stood up. All these symptoms vanished at once when I lay down flat." As spinal anesthetics became more common, it was observed that traumatic spinal taps were associated with a

lower incidence of headaches. Dr. Anthony Di Giovanni was the first to develop the modern technique of the epidural blood patch using 10 cc of autologous blood. When he presented his data at an annual meeting of the American Society of Anesthesiology in the 1960s, he was criticized by John Bonica for injecting a culture medium into the epidural space. Epidural blood patches are now the gold standard for treating postdural puncture headaches.[23]

Prevention

In our experience, the most common cause of a "wet tap" is an unrecognized blood clot obstructing the lumen of the Tuohy needle. When a clot or tissue obstructs the lumen of the needle, it is impossible to appreciate a loss of resistance. If blood drips back out of the hub of the Tuohy needle during placement, the implanter should stop, flush, and completely withdraw the needle to be certain that it is patent before proceeding. Lateral fluoroscopic imaging can also alert the implanter as to when the tip of the Tuohy needle is nearing the ligamentum flavum.

What to Do If You Get a Wet Tap

Opinions vary as to whether the procedure should continue or be aborted in the case of a dural puncture. The majority of dural rents are made with the Tuohy needle, although it is possible to tear the dura while placing a lead or guidewire. Some would advocate proceeding by removing the needle and reapproaching at a different level or on the opposite side. However, moving forward with the procedure following a dural puncture can be risky. Dural tears in the setting of SCS and lead placement can be more complicated than those encountered during routine epidural catheter placement. The 14-gauge Tuohy needle used for SCS procedures can leave a large defect in the dura, resulting in a persistent CSF leak. If a dural puncture occurs at the time of permanent implantation, the CSF will follow the path of least resistance. This can result in CSF flooding the epidural space and changing the conductance pattern, making lead placement difficult and less accurate. The CSF can also track along the course of the lead back to the midline pocket, forming a CSF hygroma. Midline hygromas are potentially hazardous because a superficial wound infection can track directly to the neuraxis via the lead, resulting in an epidural abscess or meningitis.

Unfortunately, there is no way to predict how a patient will respond to a dural puncture. Patients may experience headache and moderate neck stiffness or a serious CSF hygroma, or they may display no symptoms at all. Managing a patient with a newly implanted system who develops a postural headache and a midline hygroma following a "wet tap" can be very troublesome and problematic. If management of these complications in a patient with a newly implanted SCS system is not desired, the operation should be aborted, the postdural puncture headache treated, and the procedure rescheduled for a later time. Postdural puncture headaches can be treated conservatively at first with hydration, caffeine, analgesics, and having the patient lie flat on his or her back. If the headache does not resolve within 2 to 3 days, an epidural blood patch should be considered.

The presentation of a midline CSF hygroma is similar to that of a seroma. The term "hygroma" is nonspecific and defined only as a cystic swelling containing a serous fluid. A CSF hygroma should be suspected if there is seroma-like swelling of the midline wound after a wet tap. If the wound is soft and not tender to the touch, it can often be observed and treated in the same manner as a seroma. If the wound is tense and painful, it should be aspirated as in the case of a seroma. The area must be prepared aseptically before aspirating to prevent bacteria from entering the wound. Aspiration may be performed under fluoroscopy to avoid damaging the leads with the needle. The aspirate should be sent for culture, sensitivity testing, and fluid analysis to rule out infection or the presence of CSF. If the laboratory analysis suggests CSF, a blood patch should be performed. If an infection is present in the midline pocket and the patient had a documented dural puncture, the SCS system must be explanted immediately because of the increased risk for meningitis. Likewise, if CSF leaks from the wound at any time, a neurosurgical consult should be considered for surgical repair of the dural tear.

If the patient looks sick, has a nonpositional headache, and is febrile, meningitis must be suspected. In a case such as this, a lumbar puncture must be performed and a neurosurgical and infectious disease consult obtained immediately.

Epidural blood patches have been successfully used to seal CSF leaks postoperatively after SCS system implantation. Based on epidural flow studies, the spread of blood in the epidural space tends to be cephalad. Studies in baboons have shown that distribution of the injectate is uneven and resembles the passage of liquid between two opposing sheets of plastic. Therefore, if possible, the blood patch should be performed at the level below the dural puncture. The patient should remain recumbent for 2 hours after the blood patch to allow for clot organization. Anecdotal evidence suggests that limiting activity and avoiding Valsalva maneuvers for the next 24 hours may help to prevent dislodging of the clot. Although 90% of patients experience immediate relief from a blood patch, the long-term efficacy ranges from 61% to 75%. The blood patch may need to be repeated if the headache recurs.[23,24] If there is evidence of a persistent CSF leak after two epidural blood patches (i.e., CSF hygroma or headache), a neurosurgical consult should be considered for repair of the dural defect, with possible placement of a lumbar drain.

Although an open surgical repair of a dural tear can be successful if the tear can be localized, it is a costly and invasive procedure with potential morbidity. Alternatively, a percutaneous epidural patch with fibrin glue may be considered. Fibrin glue or sealant is a preparation of thrombin, cryoprecipitate, and calcium chloride that replicates blood coagulation to form a gel. One formulation involves injection of the contents of two syringes in equal measure—a 5-mL syringe containing a mixture of thrombin and calcium chloride, and another 5-mL syringe containing cryoprecipitate. Each syringe is attached to a Y tubing, and approximately 2 cc from each syringe (4 cc total, or stop if patient experiences pain or pressure on injection) is injected into the epidural space through an 18-gauge Tuohy needle. A fibrin clot is formed within 10 to 20 seconds of injection. There have been several case reports of successful treatment of persistent CSF leaks using 3 to 4 mL of fibrin glue injected into the epidural space with permanent resolution of headache symptoms after failed response to epidural blood patches. We have successfully treated a patient using fibrin glue after failure of two epidural blood patches. Patients must be informed that there is a risk for permanent nerve damage and that the alternative approach would entail neurosurgical repair. There is scant literature on which to base a firm recommendation. The risk for neurologic injury or allergic reaction to fibrin glue is unknown.[25,26]

Dehiscence

Wound dehiscence—the partial or complete separation of one or more layers of the surgical wound—is among the most dreaded complications encountered by surgeons. Wound dehiscence occurs in 1% to 3% of patients after abdominal surgery. Wounds will most often dehisce between 5 and 8 days after the procedure during the "lag phase," when the wound is at its weakest. Wound separation is more common in patients with diabetes, uremia, immunosuppression, cancer, or obesity and in patients who smoke or are taking corticosteroids. In the absence of patient risk factors, infection, or fluid distention, wound separation generally is the result of poor wound closure. In the case of suboptimal wound closure, dehiscence can be caused by ischemia from too much tension on the sutures or on the wound itself. Using sutures that are not strong enough or failure to close sufficient layers also contributes to wound dehiscence. Fascial layers provide strength to the healing wound. When fascial separation occurs, the wound dehisces. Most wounds separate when sutures tear through fascia. This problem can be avoided by careful wound handling and proper suture selection and technique. It is important to accurately approximate each layer and place deep sutures no more than 1 cm apart.

If wound dehiscence occurs and there is no evidence of infection, the patient can often be returned to the operating room for irrigation and reclosure. However, if the dehiscence is caused by infection, the system must be explanted.[18,21]

Perforated Viscus: Tunneling

Any patient who develops abdominal pain, hypotension, or shortness of breath should have an emergent surgical evaluation for possible pneumothorax or perforated viscus secondary to tunneling. A baseline CBC, chem panel, and a chest and upright abdominal x-ray must be obtained to rule out pneumothorax or perforated viscus. As noted in Chapter 9, it is imperative that the tip of the tunneling tool remains in the subcutaneous tissue by placing the nondominant hand on the skin over the location of the tunneling tool to determine depth during the entire pass.

Cord Injury and Nerve Damage

As the number of pain specialists performing injections has grown in the last 15 years, the number of claims associated with chronic pain management has also increased; they accounted for 10% of all claims in the 1990s. Malpractice claims were lower in chronic pain management than in surgical or obstetric anesthesia from 1970 to 1989, yet the amount of payment per incident was the same during the 1990s. Nerve injury and pneumothorax were most commonly associated with pain management malpractice claims, and epidural steroid injections accounted for 40% of all malpractice claims. Severe injuries, resulting in brain damage or death, occurred after epidural steroid injections and also with the management of implanted devices.

Recently, 13 cases occurring over a 3-year period that resulted in arachnoiditis, paralysis, anoxic brain injury, or death following cervical epidural steroid injections were reviewed from a malpractice insurer's database.[27] Cord trauma and paralysis occurred in 7 of the 13 cases, respiratory arrest resulting in anoxic brain damage or death occurred in 3 of the cases, and cord infarction and epidural hematoma each occurred in 1 patient. Another closed claim analysis of pain-related complications reported that 114 of 276 were secondary to epidural steroid blocks. Unfortunately, data regarding total complications and total procedures performed are lacking and a percentage risk factor is therefore unobtainable.

SCS procedures have much in common with epidural injections and catheter placement. Although no particular anesthetics or techniques are associated with an increased risk of neurologic

trauma, certain patterns have emerged from the closed claims analysis that may help implanters avoid neurologic injury.

An occurrence consistently associated with subsequent neural injury is sudden movement or jerking by the patient during the procedure and complaints of sudden onset of severe pain. This contrasts with the usual patient, who normally complains only of increased pressure or moderate discomfort. If a patient moves or jerks suddenly or complains of severe pain or paresthesia, the needle should immediately be removed and the patient reassessed before proceeding. The potential risks of continuing after a documented dural puncture caused by sudden patient movement should be carefully considered, as previously discussed. Firm needle control can reduce the risk of inadvertently advancing the needle if the patient jerks. A useful technique is to grasp the needle firmly with the left thumb and index finger where it enters the skin, while simultaneously resting the heel of the left hand on the patient. Thus, if the patient moves, the left hand and needle will move in concert with the patient rather than the needle unintentionally advancing as the patient jerks upward. The needle should be advanced slowly so that the patient is able to report any adverse symptoms.[27]

Sedation

The spectrum of care is broad regarding the use of sedation during epidural injection procedures. Individual implanters should decide when and how much sedation to administer. We believe that when the Tuohy needle and leads are being placed, sedation should be light for three reasons. First, a deeply sedated patient will not be able to respond to painful stimuli that can warn the implanter that the needle or lead may be doing harm. Second, a patient who is sedated to the point of somnolence may jerk to awareness and move unexpectedly. Administering a small amount of anxiolytic is helpful in calming a nervous patient, but not to the point of somnolence or sleep. Third, a sleepy patient will not be able to participate fully at the time of lead testing, possibly resulting in suboptimal lead placement.

Stenosis

Spinal stenosis and other epidural pathologies can only be diagnosed by imaging studies. After reviewing sagittal and axial magnetic resonance imaging scans, radiologists can diagnose central canal stenosis. The diagnosis must be ruled out because subclinical stenosis may result in frank myelopathy when a space-occupying lead is placed in the epidural space. In the cervical spine, the midsagittal diameter is used to diagnose stenosis. An anteroposterior (AP) diameter of less than 14 mm is cause for concern and a neuroradiologist should be consulted before proceeding with a trial. An AP diameter of less than 10 mm in the cervical spine is a contraindication to the placement of a percutaneous epidural stimulator lead. Spinal stenosis must not be present prior to proceeding.

A retrospective study published in 1996 reported an incidence of temporary paralysis of 1.8% and a 4.2% incidence of multidermatomal allodynia following placement of SCS systems in 625 patients over 12 years. Half of the patients who suffered myelopathic complications, as evidenced by upper motor neuron and posterior column signs, were awake at the time of the intraoperative onset of the deficit. Awake patients reported pain following a "specific surgical action," followed by myelopathy within 5 to 10 minutes. Neural injury was also found to be more frequent in patients undergoing laminectomy lead placement than percutaneous lead placement. As suggested by the author of the study, this relatively high percentage of cord injury may have resulted from ischemia at the time of surgery. We believe that undiagnosed spinal stenosis could have contributed to the poor outcomes.[28]

The following suggestions are helpful in minimizing neuraxial complications:[8,27]

1. Preoperatively rule out stenosis with imaging studies.
2. Know where the needle is by frequently verifying depth via lateral fluoroscopy.
3. Confirm that the Tuohy needle is patent.
4. The patient should not be overly sedated during needle and lead placement.
5. The Tuohy needle should be advanced by pinching the needle close to the skin entry point with the index finger and thumb of the left hand. The heel of the left hand should be placed on the patient's back so that if the patient moves unexpectedly, the left hand and needle will move with the patient as a unit. The implanter should never advance the needle with his or her hand suspended and out of direct contact with the patient.
6. A neurosurgeon should be asked to place a paddle lead if there is scar tissue or a previous laminectomy surgery in the path of the anticipated lead placement.
7. Because the ligamentum flavum frequently fails to fuse in the upper thoracic spine, localization of the epidural space using a loss-of-resistance technique may be more difficult.

Hardware Malfunction

SCS technology has advanced significantly in the last 25 years. Although SCS systems in general and IPGs in particular are very reliable, failures can occur from various causes. Although failures can usually be corrected on an elective basis using minimally invasive surgery, they should not be trivialized. Complications are expensive, disrupt therapy, and expose patients to additional risks. A retrospective study published in 2006 reviewed hardware failures in SCS systems placed in 289 patients at the Cleveland Clinic between 1998 and 2002. Over the period of the study, 46% of the patients required at least one revision, not including depleted battery replacements;

22.5% required more than one revision. Of these revisions, none were caused by IPG failure.[5]

When hardware failures occur, they are almost invariably caused by lead problems. The Cleveland Clinic found that failures in SCS systems employing percutaneous-type leads resulted from lead migration (12%), poor coverage (12.3%), and breakage (6.8%). In the study, infection was considered a hardware failure and was seen in 3.3% of the leads that were placed. As might be expected, the rates of lead migration and fractures were 25% and 40%, respectively, and they were more commonly seen with cervical lead placement than with thoracic lead placement. Poor coverage, however, was 27% more common with thoracic lead placement. The review unexpectedly found that surgical leads had higher incidences of infection, lead migration, and lead breakage than percutaneous leads.

As anchoring technology improves, lead migration and breakage are expected to become less frequent. Improved IPG capabilities will no doubt lead to improved ability to recapture lost coverage, which can often be the result of epidural fibrosis and micromigration.[5]

We have found IPGs to be exceedingly reliable; it is highly unusual for an IPG to fail. In our combined experience at the University of California Davis, we have had only a single IPG failure in a patient following emergent cardioversion after an episode of ventricular tachycardia. After successful cardioversion, the IPG failed to function and was replaced after it was determined that the patient would not require a pacemaker. The patient has continued to do well since the IPG replacement. Some rechargeable IPGs have been constructed to resist short-circuit damage that may result from extraneous electrical current, as may be caused by electrocautery or cardioversion. If there is a significant possibility that the patient may need cardioversion or surgery requiring electrocautery, selection of a battery that is manufactured to resist circuit damage caused by such devices is recommended. The manufacturer should be consulted to determine the best choice for the patient.

Finally, there is a single case report in the literature—from 1993—of interference between a unipolar pacemaker and a unipolar SCS. In 1998, the same author published a case report demonstrating the safe use of a dual-pacing, dual-sensing, dual-mode pacemaker in a patient with implanted quadripolar SCS electrodes. A recent poster session presented five patients with SCS and pacemakers who experienced no electrical interference between the two units. The manufacturers of both devices should be contacted prior to SCS implantation in patients with pacemakers.[29,30]

REFERENCES

1. Kohn LT, Corrigan JM, Donaldson MS. *To err is human: building a safer health system.* Washington, DC: National Press, 1999.
2. American Health Quality Association. American Journal of Surgery: *QIO national collaborative cuts surgical infection rates.*

June 23, 2005. Available at: http://ahqa.newc.com/pub/connections/162_696_5223.cfm#amer

3. Stojanovic MP, Abdi S. Spinal cord stimulation. *Pain Physician* 2002;5:156–66.

4. Cameron T. Safety and efficacy of spinal cord stimulation for the treatment of chronic pain: a 20-year literature review. *J Neurosurg* 2004;100(3):254–67.

5. Rosenow JM, Stanton-Hicks M, Rezai AR, et al. Failure modes of SCS hardware. *J Neurosurg* 2006;5:183–90.

6. American Society of Anesthesiologists House of Delegates. *ASA standards for basic anesthetic monitoring.* Approved October 21 1986; amended October 25, 2005.

7. Weinberg G. Lipid infusion resuscitation for local anesthetic toxicity: proof of clinical efficacy. *Anesthesiology* 2006;105(1):7–8.

8. Miller RD. *Miller's anesthesia,* 6th ed. New York: Elsevier, 2005.

9. Darouiche RO. Treatment of infections associated with surgical implants. *N Engl J Med* 2004;350:1422–9.

10. Rathmell JP, Lake T, Ramundo MB. Infectious risks of chronic pain treatments: injection therapy, surgical implants, and intradiscal techniques. *Reg Anesth Pain Med* 2006;31(4):346–52.

11. Peterson JJ. Postoperative Infection. *Rad Clin North Am* 2006;44(3):439–50.

12. Hunt TK. Wound healing: forms of healing. In: Doherty GM, Way LW, eds. *Current surgical diagnosis and treatment,* 12th ed. Norwalk, CT: Appleton & Lange, 2006.

13. Franzini A, Ferroli P, Marras C, et al. Huge epidural hematoma after surgery for spinal cord stimulation. *Acta Neurochir* 2005;147(5):565–7.

14. Smith BE. Epidural anesthesia/analgesia and coronary artery bypass surgery utilizing extracorporeal circulation. *Chest* 2005;128:1097–9.

15. Jaffer AK, Brotman DJ, Chukwumerije N. When patients on warfarin need surgery. *Cleve Clin J Med* 2003;701(1):973–84.

16. Horlocker TT. Low molecular weight heparin and neuraxial anesthesia. *Thrombosis Res* 2001;101(1):141–54.

17. Rainov NG, Holzhausen HJ, Burkert W. Complete disappearance of giant intracranial germinoma after irradiation. *Neurosurg Rev* 1995;18(4):285–92.

18. Mulholland MW, Doherty GM. *Complications in surgery.* Philadelphia: Lippincott Williams & Wilkins. 2006.

19. Mackenzie AR, Laing RB, Smith CC, et al. Spinal epidural abscess: the importance of early diagnosis and treatment. *J Neurol Neurosurg Psychiatry* 1998;65:209–12.

20. Huff JS. Spinal epidural abscess. *eMedicine.* January 17, 2007. Available at: http://www.emedicine.com/neuro/topic349.htm. Accessed June 19, 2007.

21. Doherty GM, Way LW, eds. *Current surgical diagnosis and treatment,* 12th ed. New York: McGraw Hill, 2006.

22. Nadkarni MS, Rangole AK, Sharma RK, et al. Influence of surgical technique on axillary seroma formation: a randomized study. *ANZ J Surg* 2007;77(5):385–9.

23. Harrington BE. Postdural puncture headache and the development of the epidural blood patch. *Reg Anesth Pain Med* 2004;29(2):136–63.

24. Hogan Q. Distribution of solution in the epidural space: examination by cryomicrotome section. *Reg Anesth Pain Med* 2002;27(2):150–6.

25. Crul BJ, Gerritse BM, van Dongen RT, et al. Epidural fibrin glue injection stops persistent postdural puncture headache. *Anesthesiology* 1999;91(2):576–7.

26. Gladstone JP, Nelson K, Patel N, et al. Spontaneous CSF leak treated with percutaneous CT-guided fibrin glue. *Neurology* 2005;64(10):1818–9.

27. Lofsky AF. Complications of cervical epidural blocks attract insurance company attention. *APSF Newsletter.* Fall 2005. Available at: http://www.apsf.org/resource_center/newsletter/2005/fall/03cervical.htm. Accessed June 19, 2008.

28. Law JD. Hypothesis about the etiology of unexplained painful myelopathy after minor trauma in the spinal canal. *Stereotact Funct Neurosurg* 1995;65(1-4):117–9.

29. Krakovsky AA. *Cardiac pacemaker and spinal cord stimulator: do they interfere?* AAPM Poster No. 104. 22nd Annual Meeting of the American Academy of Pain Medicine, February 23, 2006.

30. Romano M, Brusa S, Grieco A, et al. Efficacy and safety of permanent cardiac DDD pacing with contemporaneous double spinal cord stimulation. *Pacing Clin Electrophysiol* 1998:21(2):465–7.

Further Reading

Dural Puncture

Burchiel KJ, Anderson VC, Brown FD, et al. Prospective, multicenter study of spinal cord stimulation for relief of chronic back and extremity pain. *Spine* 1996;21(23):2786–94.

Eldrige JS, Weingarten TN, Rho RH. Management of cerebral spinal fluid leak complicating spinal cord stimulator implantation. *Pain Pract* 2006;6(4):285–8.

Forouzanfar T, Kemler MA, Weber WE, et al. Spinal cord stimulation in complex regional pain syndrome: cervical and lumbar devices are comparably effective. *Br J Anaesth* 2004;92(3):348–53.

Kemler MA, Barendse GA, van Kleef M, et al. Spinal cord stimulation in patients with chronic reflex sympathetic dystrophy. *N Engl J Med* 2000;343(9):618–24.

Kumar K, Toth C, Nath RK, et al. Epidural spinal cord stimulation for treatment of chronic pain—some predictors of success. A 15-year experience. *Surg Neurol* 1998;50(2):110–20.

Epidural Hematoma

Abejón D, Reig E, del Pozo C, et al. Dual spinal cord stimulation for complex pain: preliminary study. *Neuromodulation* 2005;8(2):105–1.

Aló KM, Redko V, Charnov J. Four year follow-up of dual electrode spinal cord stimulation for chronic pain. *Neuromodulation* 2002;5(2):79–99.

Aló KM, Yland MJ, Charnov JH, et al. Multiple program spinal cord stimulation in the treatment of chronic pain: follow-up of multiple program SCS. *Neuromodulation* 1999;2(4):266–72.

Barolat G. Experience with 509 plate electrodes implanted epidurally from C1 to L1. *Stereotact Funct Neurosurg* 1993;61(2):60–79.

Bennett DS, Aló KM, Oakley J, et al. Spinal cord stimulation for complex regional pain syndrome I (RSD). A retrospective multicenter experience from 1995-1998 of 101 patients. *Neuromodulation* 1999;2(3):202-10.

Franzini A, Ferroli P, Marras C, et al. Huge epidural hematoma after surgery for spinal cord stimulation. *Acta Neurochir (Wien)* 2005;147(5):565–7.

Kumar K, Hunter G, Demeria D. Spinal cord stimulation in treatment of chronic benign pain: challenges in treatment planning and present status, a 22-year experience. *Neurosurgery* 2006; 58(3):481–96.

Kumar K, Toth C, Nath RK, et al. Epidural spinal cord stimulation for treatment of chronic pain—some predictors of success. A 15-year experience. *Surg Neurol* 1998;50(2):110–20.

Kumar K, Wilson JR, Taylor RS, Gupta S. Complications of spinal cord stimulation, suggestions to improve outcome, and financial impact. *J Neurosurg Spine* 2006;5(3):191–203.

Meglio M, Cioni B, Rossi GF. Spinal cord stimulation in management of chronic pain. A 9-year experience. *J Neurosurg* 1989;70(4): 519–24.

Shealy CN. Dorsal column stimulation: optimization of application. *Surg Neurol* 1975;4(1):142–5.

Slavin KV, Burchiel KJ, Anderson VC, et al. Efficacy of transverse tripolar stimulation for relief of chronic low back pain: results of a single center. *Stereotact Funct Neurosurg* 1999;73(1-4): 126–30.

Infection

Abejón D, Reig E, del Pozo C, et al. Dual spinal cord stimulation for complex pain: preliminary study. *Neuromodulation* 2005;8(2): 105–1.

Aló KM, Redko V, Charnov J. Four year follow-up of dual electrode spinal cord stimulation for chronic pain. *Neuromodulation* 2002;5(2):79–99.

Aló KM, Yland MJ, Charnov JH, et al. Multiple program spinal cord stimulation in the treatment of chronic pain: follow-up of multiple program SCS. *Neuromodulation* 1999;2(4):266–72.

Arxer A, Busquets C, Vilaplana J, et al. Subacute epidural abscess after spinal cord stimulation implantation [letter]. *Eur J Anesthesiol* 2003;20:753–9.

Barolat G. Experience with 509 plate electrodes implanted epidurally from C1 to L1. *Stereotact Funct Neurosurg* 1993;61(2):60–79.

Barolat G, Schwartzman R, Woo R. Epidural spinal cord stimulation in the management of reflex sympathetic dystrophy. *Stereotact Funct Neurosurg* 1989;53(1):29–39.

Bennett DS, Aló KM, Oakley J, et al. Spinal cord stimulation for complex regional pain syndrome I (RSD). A retrospective multicenter experience from 1995–1998 of 101 patients. *Neuromodulation* 1999;2(3):202–10.

Blond S, Armignies P, Parker F, et al. Chronic sciatalgia caused by sensitive deafferentiation following surgery for lumbar disk hernia: clinical and therapeutic aspects. Apropos of 110 patients [in French]. *Neurochirurgie* 1991;37(2):86–95.

Burchiel KJ, Anderson VC, Brown FD, et al. Prospective, multicenter study of spinal cord stimulation for relief of chronic back and extremity pain. *Spine* 1996;21(23):2786–94.

de la Porte C, Siegfried J. Lumbosacral spinal fibrosis (spinal arachnoiditis). Its diagnosis and treatment by spinal cord stimulation. *Spine* 1983;8(6):593–603.

De Mulder PA, te Rijdt B, Veeckmans G, et al. Evaluation of a dual quadripolar surgically implanted spinal cord stimulation lead for failed back surgery patients with chronic low back and leg pain. *Neuromodulation* 2005;8(4):219–24.

Follett KA, Boortz-Marx RL, Drake JM, et al. Prevention and management of intrathecal drug delivery and spinal cord stimulation system infections. *Anesthesiology* 2004;100(6):1582–94.

Forouzanfar T, Kemler MA, Weber WE, et al. Spinal cord stimulation in complex regional pain syndrome: cervical and lumbar devices are comparably effective. *Br J Anaesth* 2004;92(3):348–53.

Kay AD, McIntyre MD, Macrae WA, et al. Spinal cord stimulation—a long-term evaluation in patients with chronic pain. *Br J Neurosurg* 2001;115(4):335–41.

Kemler MA, Barendse GA, van Kleef M, et al. Electrical spinal cord stimulation in reflex sympathetic dystrophy: retrospective analysis of 23 patients. *J Neurosurg* 1999;90(1 Suppl):79–83.

Kumar A, Felderhof C, Eljamel MS. Spinal cord stimulation for the treatment of refractory unilateral limb pain syndromes. *Stereotact Funct Neurosurg* 2003;81(1-4):70–4.

Kumar K, Hunter G, Demeria D. Spinal cord stimulation in treatment of chronic benign pain: challenges in treatment planning and present status, a 22-year experience. *Neurosurgery* 2006; 58(3):481–96.

Kumar K, Malik S, Demeria D. Treatment of chronic pain with spinal cord stimulation versus alternative therapies: cost-effectiveness analysis. *Neurosurgery* 2002;51(1):106–15.

Kumar K, Nath R, Wyant GM. Treatment of chronic pain by epidural spinal cord stimulation: a 10-year experience. *J Neurosurg* 1991; 75(3):402–7.

Kumar K, Toth C. The role of spinal cord stimulation in the treatment of chronic pain postlaminectomy. *Curr Pain Headache Rep* 1998;2:85–92.

Kumar K, Toth C, Nath RK, et al. Epidural spinal cord stimulation for treatment of chronic pain—some predictors of success. A 15-year experience. *Surg Neurol* 1998;50(2):110–20.

Kumar K, Wilson JR, Taylor RS, Gupta S. Complications of spinal cord stimulation, suggestions to improve outcome, and financial impact. *J Neurosurg Spine* 2006;5(3):191–203.

Lang P. The treatment of chronic pain by epidural spinal cord stimulation—a 15-year follow-up: present status. *Axon* 1997; 71–3.

Leclercq TA, Russo E. Epidural stimulation for pain control [in French]. *Neurochirurgie* 1981;27(2):125–8.

Leveque JC, Villavicencio AT, Bulsara KR, et al. Spinal cord stimulation for failed back surgery syndrome. *Neuromodulation* 2001; 4(1):1–9.

May MS, Banks C, Thomson SJ. A retrospective, long-term, third-party follow-up of patients considered for spinal cord stimulation. *Neuromodulation* 2002;5(3):137–44.

Meglio M, Cioni B, Rossi GF. Spinal cord stimulation in management of chronic pain. A 9-year experience. *J Neurosurg* 1989;70(4): 519–24.

Meglio M, Cioni B, Visocchi M, et al. Spinal cord stimulation in low back and leg pain. *Stereotact Funct Neurosurg* 1994;62 (1–4):263–6.

Ohnmeiss DD, Rashbaum RF, Bogdanffy GM. Prospective outcome evaluation of spinal cord stimulation in patients with intractable leg pain. *Spine* 1996;1;21(11):1344–50.

Quigley DG, Arnold J, Eldridge PR, et al. Long-term outcome of spinal cord stimulation and hardware complications. *Stereotact Funct Neurosurg* 2003;81(1–4):50–63.

Renard VM, North RB. Prevention of percutaneous electrode migration in spinal cord stimulation by a modification of the standard implantation technique. *J Neurosurg Spine* 2006;4(4):300–3.

Rosenow JM, Stanton-Hicks M, Rezai AR, et al. Failure modes of spinal cord stimulation hardware. *J Neurosurg Spine* 2006;5: 183–90.

Segal R, Stacey BR, Rudy TE, et al. Spinal cord stimulation revisited. *Neurol Res* 1998;20(5):391–6.

Shealy CN. Dorsal column stimulation: optimization of application. *Surg Neurol* 1975;4(1):142–5.

Siegfried J, Lazorthes Y. Long-term follow-up of dorsal cord stimulation for chronic pain syndrome after multiple lumbar operations. *Appl Neurophysiol* 1982;45:201–4.

Simpson BA. Spinal cord stimulation in 60 cases of intractable pain. *J Neurol Neurosurg Psychiatry* 1991;54(3):196–9.

Simpson BA, Bassett G, Davies K, et al. Cervical spinal cord stimulation for pain: a report on 41 patients. *Neuromodulation* 2003; 6(1):20–6.

Slavin KV, Burchiel KJ, Anderson VC, et al. Efficacy of transverse tripolar stimulation for relief of chronic low back pain: results of a single center. *Stereotact Funct Neurosurg* 1999;73(1-4): 126–30.

Sundaraj SR, Johnstone C, Noore F, et al. Spinal cord stimulation: a seven-year audit. *J Clin Neurosci* 2005;12(3):264–70.

Vall de Cabres V, Solans Laque R, Pigrau Sarrallach C, et al. Psoas abscess due to an epidural spinal cord stimulation catheter. *Scand J Infect Dis* 1992;24(1):119.

van Buyten J-P, van Zundert J, Vueghs P, et al. Efficacy of spinal cord stimulation: 10 years of experience in a pain centre in Belgium. *Eur J Pain* 2001;5(3):299–307.

Villavicencio AT, Leveque JC, Rubin L, et al. Laminectomy versus percutaneous electrode placement for spinal cord stimulation. *Neurosurgery* 2000;46(2):399–405.

Wound Breakdown, Dehiscence

Blond S, Armignies P, Parker F, et al. Chronic sciatalgia caused by sensitive deafferentiation following surgery for lumbar disk hernia: clinical and therapeutic aspects. Apropos of 110 patients [in French]. *Neurochirurgie* 1991;37(2):86–95.

de la Porte C, Siegfried J. Lumbosacral spinal fibrosis (spinal arachnoiditis). Its diagnosis and treatment by spinal cord stimulation. *Spine* 1983;8(6):593–603.

Electrode Migration

Abejón D, Reig E, del Pozo C, et al. Dual spinal cord stimulation for complex pain: preliminary study. *Neuromodulation* 2005;8(2): 105–1.

Aló KM, Redko V, Charnov J. Four year follow-up of dual electrode spinal cord stimulation for chronic pain. *Neuromodulation* 2002;5(2):79–99.

Aló KM, Yland MJ, Charnov JH, et al. Multiple program spinal cord stimulation in the treatment of chronic pain: follow-up of multiple program SCS. *Neuromodulation* 1999;2(4):266–72.

Barolat G. Experience with 509 plate electrodes implanted epidurally from C1 to L1. *Stereotact Funct Neurosurg* 1993;61(2):60–79.

Barolat G, Schwartzman R, Woo R. Epidural spinal cord stimulation in the management of reflex sympathetic dystrophy. *Stereotact Funct Neurosurg* 1989;53(1):29–39.

Blond S, Armignies P, Parker F, et al. Chronic sciatalgia caused by sensitive deafferentiation following surgery for lumbar disk hernia: clinical and therapeutic aspects. Apropos of 110 patients [in French]. *Neurochirurgie* 1991;37(2):86–95.

Broseta J, Roldan P, Gonzalez-Darder J, et al. Chronic epidural dorsal column stimulation in the treatment of causalgic pain. *Appl Neurophysiol* 1982;45:190–4.

Budd K. Spinal cord stimulation: cost–benefit study. *Neuromodulation* 2002;5(2):75–8.

Burchiel KJ, Anderson VC, Brown FD, et al. Prospective, multicenter study of spinal cord stimulation for relief of chronic back and extremity pain. *Spine* 1996;21(23):2786–94.

Burton AW, Fukshansky M, Brown J, et al. Refractory insomnia in a patient with spinal cord stimulator lead migration. *Neuromodulation* 2004;7(4):242–5.

de la Porte C, Siegfried J. Lumbosacral spinal fibrosis (spinal arachnoiditis). Its diagnosis and treatment by spinal cord stimulation. *Spine* 1983;8(6):593–603.

Forouzanfar T, Kemler MA, Weber WE, et al. Spinal cord stimulation in complex regional pain syndrome: cervical and lumbar devices are comparably effective. *Br J Anaesth* 2004;92(3):348–53.

Kavar B, Rosenfeld JV, Hutchinson A. The efficacy of spinal cord stimulation for chronic pain. *J Clin Neurosci* 2000;7(5): 409–13.

Kay AD, McIntyre MD, Macrae WA, et al. Spinal cord stimulation—a long-term evaluation in patients with chronic pain. *Br J Neurosurg* 2001;15(4):335–41.

Kumar A, Felderhof C, Eljamel MS. Spinal cord stimulation for the treatment of refractory unilateral limb pain syndromes. *Stereotact Funct Neurosurg* 2003;81(1-4):70–4.

Kumar K, Hunter G, Demeria D. Spinal cord stimulation in treatment of chronic benign pain: challenges in treatment planning and present status, a 22-year experience. *Neurosurgery* 2006; 58(3):481–96.

Kumar K, Malik S, Demeria D. Treatment of chronic pain with spinal cord stimulation versus alternative therapies: cost-effectiveness analysis. *Neurosurgery* 2002;51(1):106–15.

Kumar K, Nath RK, Toth C. Spinal cord stimulation is effective in the management of reflex sympathetic dystrophy. *Neurosurgery* 1997;40(3):503–8.

Kumar K, Nath R, Wyant GM. Treatment of chronic pain by epidural spinal cord stimulation: a 10-year experience. *J Neurosurg* 1991; 75(3):402–7.

Kumar K, Toth C. The role of spinal cord stimulation in the treatment of chronic pain postlaminectomy. *Curr Pain Headache Rep* 1998;2:85–92.

Kumar K, Toth C, Nath RK, et al. Epidural spinal cord stimulation for treatment of chronic pain—some predictors of success. A 15-year experience. *Surg Neurol* 1998;50(2):110–20.

Lang P. The treatment of chronic pain by epidural spinal cord stimulation—a 15-year follow-up: present status. *Axon* 1997;71–3.

Leclercq TA. Electrode migration in epidural stimulation: comparison between singles electrode and four electrode programmable leads. *Pain* 1984;20(Suppl 2):78.

Leclercq TA, Russo E. Epidural stimulation for pain control [in French]. *Neurochirurgie* 1981;27(2):125–8.

Leveque JC, Villavicencio AT, Bulsara KR, et al. Spinal cord stimulation for failed back surgery syndrome. *Neuromodulation* 2001; 4(1):1–9.

May MS, Banks C, Thomson SJ. A retrospective, long-term, third-party follow-up of patients considered for spinal cord stimulation. *Neuromodulation* 2002;5(3):137–44.

Meglio M, Cioni B, Rossi GF. Spinal cord stimulation in management of chronic pain. A 9-year experience. *J Neurosurg* 1989;70(4): 519–24.

Meglio M, Cioni B, Visocchi M, et al. Spinal cord stimulation in low back and leg pain. *Stereotact Funct Neurosurg* 1994;62(1-4):263–6.

North RB, Kidd DH, Olin J, et al. Spinal cord stimulation for axial low back pain: a prospective, controlled trial comparing dual with single percutaneous electrodes. *Spine* 2005;30(12):1412–8.

North RB, Kidd DH, Zahurak M, et al. Spinal cord stimulation for chronic, intractable pain: experience over two decades. *Neurosurgery* 1993;32(3):384–94.

Ohnmeiss DD, Rashbaum RF, Bogdanffy GM. Prospective outcome evaluation of spinal cord stimulation in patients with intractable leg pain. *Spine* 1996;21(11):1344–50.

Quigley DG, Arnold J, Eldridge PR, et al. Long-term outcome of spinal cord stimulation and hardware complications. *Stereotact Funct Neurosurg* 2003;81(1-4):50–6.

Racz GB, McCarron RF, Talboys P. Percutaneous dorsal column stimulator for chronic pain control. *Spine* 1989;14(1):1–4.

Renard VM, North RB. Prevention of percutaneous electrode migration in spinal cord stimulation by a modification of the standard implantation technique. *J Neurosurg Spine* 2006;4(4):300–3.

Rosenow JM, Stanton-Hicks M, Rezai AR, et al. Failure modes of spinal cord stimulation hardware. *J Neurosurg Spine* 2006;5:183–90.

Siegfried J, Lazorthes Y. Long-term follow-up of dorsal cord stimulation for chronic pain syndrome after multiple lumbar operations. *Appl Neurophysiol* 1982;45:201–4.

Simpson BA, Bassett G, Davies K, et al. Cervical spinal cord stimulation for pain: a report on 41 patients. *Neuromodulation* 2003;6(1):20–6.

Spiegelmann R, Friedman WA. Spinal cord stimulation: a contemporary series. *Neurosurgery* 1991;28(1):65–70.

Sundaraj SR, Johnstone C, Noore F, et al. Spinal cord stimulation: a seven-year audit. *J Clin Neurosci* 2005;12(3):264–70.

Tseng SH. Treatment of chronic pain by spinal cord stimulation. *J Formos Med Assoc* 2000;99(3):267–71.

Vallejo R, Kramer J, Benyamin R. Neuromodulation of the cervical spinal cord in the treatment of chronic intractable neck and upper extremity pain: a case series and review of the literature. *Pain Physician* 2007;10(2):305–11.

van Buyten J-P, van Zundert J, Vueghs P, et al. Efficacy of spinal cord stimulation: 10 years of experience in a pain centre in Belgium. *Eur J Pain* 2001;5(3):299–307.

Device Failure

Aló KM, Redko V, Charnov J. Four-year follow-up of dual electrode spinal cord stimulation for chronic pain. *Neuromodulation* 2002;5(2):79–99.

Barolat G. Experience with 509 plate electrodes implanted epidurally from C1 to L1. *Stereotact Funct Neurosurg* 1993;61(2):60–79.

Barolat G, Schwartzman R, Woo R. Epidural spinal cord stimulation in the management of reflex sympathetic dystrophy. *Stereotact Funct Neurosurg* 1989;53(1):29–39.

Blond S, Armignies P, Parker F, et al. Chronic sciatalgia caused by sensitive deafferentiation following surgery for lumbar disk hernia: clinical and therapeutic aspects. Apropos of 110 patients [in French]. *Neurochirurgie* 1991;37(2):86–95.

Broseta J, Roldan P, Gonzalez-Darder J, et al. Chronic epidural dorsal column stimulation in the treatment of causalgic pain. *Appl Neurophysiol* 1982;45:190–4.

Burchiel KJ, Anderson VC, Brown FD, et al. Prospective, multicenter study of spinal cord stimulation for relief of chronic back and extremity pain. *Spine* 1996;21(23):2786–94.

De Andres J, Quiroz C, Villanueva V, et al. Patient satisfaction with spinal cord stimulation for failed back surgery syndrome [in Spanish]. *Rev Esp Anestesiol Reanim* 2007;54(1):17–22.

de la Porte C, Siegfried J. Lumbosacral spinal fibrosis (spinal arachnoiditis). Its diagnosis and treatment by spinal cord stimulation. *Spine* 1983;8(6):593–603.

Forouzanfar T, Kemler MA, Weber WE, et al. Spinal cord stimulation in complex regional pain syndrome: cervical and lumbar devices are comparably effective. *Br J Anaesth* 2004;92(3):348–53.

Heidecke V, Rainov NG, Burkert W. Hardware failures in spinal cord stimulation for failed back surgery syndrome. *Neuromodulation* 2000;3(1):27–30.

Kay AD, McIntyre MD, Macrae WA, et al. Spinal cord stimulation—a long-term evaluation in patients with chronic pain. *Br J Neurosurg* 2001;15(4):335–41.

Kumar A, Felderhof C, Eljamel MS. Spinal cord stimulation for the treatment of refractory unilateral limb pain syndromes. *Stereotact Funct Neurosurg* 2003;81(1-4):70–4.

Kumar K, Hunter G, Demeria D. Spinal cord stimulation in treatment of chronic benign pain: challenges in treatment planning and present status, a 22-year experience. *Neurosurgery* 2006;58(3):481–96.

Kumar K, Malik S, Demeria D. Treatment of chronic pain with spinal cord stimulation versus alternative therapies: cost-effectiveness analysis. *Neurosurgery* 2002;51(1):106–15.

Kumar K, Nath TK, Toth C. Spinal cord stimulation is effective in the management of reflex sympathetic dystrophy. *Neurosurgery* 1997;40(3):503–8.

Kumar K, Nath R, Wyant GM. Treatment of chronic pain by epidural spinal cord stimulation: a 10-year experience. *J Neurosurg* 1991;75(3):402–7.

Kumar K, Toth C. The role of spinal cord stimulation in the treatment of chronic pain postlaminectomy. *Curr Pain Headache Rep* 1998;2:85–92.

Kumar K, Toth C, Nath RK, Laing P. Epidural spinal cord stimulation for treatment of chronic pain—some predictors of success. A 15-year experience. *Surg Neurol* 1998;50(2):110–20.

Kumar K, Wilson JR, Taylor RS, et al. Complications of spinal cord stimulation, suggestions to improve outcome, and financial impact. *J Neurosurg Spine* 2006;5(3):191–203.

Lang P. The treatment of chronic pain by epidural spinal cord stimulation—a 15-year follow-up: present status. *Axon* 1997;71–3.

Leveque JC, Villavicencio AT, Bulsara KR, et al. Spinal cord stimulation for failed back surgery syndrome. *Neuromodulation* 2001;4(1):1–9.

May MS, Banks C, Thomson SJ. A retrospective, long-term, third-party follow-up of patients considered for spinal cord stimulation. *Neuromodulation* 2002;5(3):137–44.

Meglio M, Cioni B, Rossi GF. Spinal cord stimulation in management of chronic pain. A 9-year experience. *J Neurosurg* 1989;70(4):519–24.

Meglio M, Cioni B, Visocchi M, et al. Spinal cord stimulation in low back and leg pain. *Stereotact Funct Neurosurg* 1994;62(1-4):263–6.

North RB, Kidd DH, Olin J, et al. Spinal cord stimulation for axial low back pain: a prospective, controlled trial comparing dual with single percutaneous electrodes. *Spine* 2005;30(12):1412–8.

North RB, Kidd DH, Zahurak M, et al. Spinal cord stimulation for chronic, intractable pain: experience over two decades. *Neurosurgery* 1993;32(3):384–94.

Quigley DG, Arnold J, Eldridge PR, et al. Long-term outcome of spinal cord stimulation and hardware complications. *Stereotact Funct Neurosurg* 2003;81(1-4):50–6.

Racz GB, McCarron RF, Talboys P. Percutaneous dorsal column stimulator for chronic pain control. *Spine* 1989;14(1):1–4.

Rosenow JM, Stanton-Hicks M, Rezai AR, et al. Failure modes of spinal cord stimulation hardware. *J Neurosurg Spine* 2006;5: 183–90.

Simpson BA, Bassett G, Davies K, et al. Cervical spinal cord stimulation for pain: a report on 41 patients. *Neuromodulation* 2003; 6(1):20–6.

Sundaraj SR, Johnstone C, Noore F, et al. Spinal cord stimulation: a seven-year audit. *J Clin Neurosci* 2005;12(3):264–70.

Vallejo R, Kramer J, Benyamin R. Neuromodulation of the cervical spinal cord in the treatment of chronic intractable neck and upper extremity pain: a case series and review of the literature. *Pain Physician* 2007;10(2):305–11.

van Buyten J-P, van Zundert J, Vueghs P, et al. Efficacy of spinal cord stimulation: 10 years of experience in a pain centre in Belgium. *Eur J Pain* 2001;5(3):299–307.

Index

Note: Page numbers followed by *f* refer to figures; page numbers followed by *t* refer to tables.